The goal of this book is

MORE VIGOROUS LIVING DURING LATER YEARS!

"You show the universal significance to all body tissues of vitamin E; anyone would be naturally interested in something that makes their body function more effectively and may even prolong life. . . .

"You have managed to put vitamin E in its proper perspective. . . ."

Letter to the Author
CHRISTOPHER COOK, M.D.
Association of Life Insurance Medical Directors of America

The author, Erwin Di Cyan, Ph.D., is a drug consultant and writer on subjects in science and health for the layman. His most recent book, which appeared in April 1972, is *Without Prescription*, published by Simon & Schuster. It is a guide to the selection and use of medicines available to the layman over the counter, without prescription. Dr. Di Cyan has been active in drug research and development for about 28 years.

VITAMIN E AND AGING

ERWIN Di CYAN, Ph.D.

Foreword by

CHRISTOPHER COOK, M.D.
Association of Life Insurance Medical Directors of America

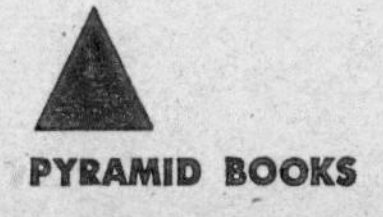

PYRAMID BOOKS • NEW YORK

VITAMIN E AND AGING

A PYRAMID BOOK

First edition, July 1972

ISBN 0–515–02761–8

Library of Congress Catalog Card Number: 72–80402

Pyramid Books are published by Pyramid Communications, Inc. Its trademarks, consisting of the word "pyramid" and the portrayal of a pyramid, are registered in the United States Patent Office.

PYRAMID COMMUNICATIONS, INC.
919 Third Avenue
New York, New York 10022, U.S.A.

Table of Contents

Foreword

CHRISTOPHER COOK, M.D.
Association of Life Insurance Medical Directors of America

Vitamin E is a fascinating substance. It is found in every tissue of the body. Why? It must be performing an essential function. The preponderance of evidence is that it protects the cells of our body against incipient destructive oxidation in the wrong places. Because of this function it is of paramount importance in determining how long the cells in our body survive and therefore how long we live.

If the cells are not protected against oxidation they burn up, and if more are destroyed than are replaced the body gradually deteriorates or ages. This process takes about 70 years. There is a strong suspicion among the eminent researchers in vitamin E from many countries of the world that vitamin E may be a key factor in slowing this process. Because they are dealing with such minute changes over such a span of time, research in this field is slow and tedious. Nonetheless, specific gains have been made, and the subject is one that looks highly promising—if the research were greatly expanded.

Nevertheless, the role of vitamin E, which has been virtually ignored, has recently risen into prominence. For example, the U.S. Food and Drug Administration (FDA), which had in the past demanded a disclaimer on the label of vitamin E products stating that the need for vitamin E in human nutrition has not been established, has now modified its position: it has conceded that there is a clear need for vitamin E in human nutrition. The fact that the FDA has not yet established the "minimum daily requirement" merely means that the minimum given amount needed daily has not been legally fixed. And that is true: there is a range, varying with different investigators from about 7 to 50 International Units (I.U.), which they believe is the daily amount needed to prevent deficiency.

In fact, the recent (1968) National Research Council's Recommended Daily Allowances, conceding that vitamin E is necessary in *human* nutrition, states that different amounts are needed by people of different ages or conditions: infants up to 1 year need 5 I.U.; children up to 6 years, 10 I.U.; children from 6 to 10 years, 15 I.U.; in older children the amounts differ with sex. The daily amounts for adults also vary with sex: men are held to need 30 I.U., women 25 I.U., but 30 I.U. is recommended for lactating and pregnant women. All amounts are daily.

In December 1971 an important conference on vitamin E was held in New York by the New York Academy of Sciences. Reflecting the renewed interest in and importance of vitamin E, that conference was devoted to basic biochemical studies. Such studies are of prime importance in determining if or how vitamin E works in various conditions for the best function of the body economy.

I believe that vitamin E slows down the process of aging, so that taking it in sufficient daily amounts can possibly make a person of 60 look, act, feel, *seem,* and *be* more like a person of 50, or a person of 70 look, act, feel, seem, and be more like a person of, say, 60. Ultimately age will catch up with the vitamin E user—but perhaps much later in the game. I believe this for good scientific reasons, which are increasingly being offered.

When I speak of aging I am not talking about the good aspects, such as increased wisdom, but the bad side of aging. Aging in medicine means deterioration. It means a slower gait, dimmer eyesight, harder breathing, shakier hands, less and less enjoyment of all the pleasures—food, talk, laughter, love, sex, sleeping, getting up, social interest, using one's brain—of life. These concomitants of aging, as considered here, are regrettable and something to be put off as long as possible.

Introduction

Age does not suddenly appear in the doorway of life. Aging is a gradual process. A few people do feel that they suddenly turned old—either through hearing catastrophic news or through their histrionic desire to splash drama all over their surroundings; but people normally do not suddenly or dramatically turn old.

The old adage has it that we begin to age from the moment of birth. By a strict construction that is true. But different organs age at a different rate. For example: baby teeth grow old and begin to fall out at about 6 years of age to be replaced by "permanent" teeth. These are the teeth that the individual has throughout his adult life. And they too deteriorate and fall out beginning perhaps in the 40s or later.

Each individual has certain behavioral traits which make up his personality. These traits begin to develop at or shortly after infancy. They mature during adolescence, are fixed in adulthood, become rigidly a part of the individual upon aging and become exaggerated during old age. For example, a young adult may be economical, as he or she matures he may be frugal, then the trait is exaggerated into niggardliness or miserliness–depending upon his socioeconomic constellation –during old age.

Similarly, physical symptoms also become exaggerated. Hence, one cannot speak of aging per se without realizing that physiological or psychological events about a person are true throughout his or her life.

Hence, when we speak of vitamin E or any other nutrient, we are dealing with events throughout life—occurring at different rates—which are merely accentuated in aging. During aging, then, the needs are much the same; merely more careful and selective nutritional and other ministrations are necessary to make up for the normal abnormality—that is, selective deterioration—which takes place as we grow in years.

Has vitamin E been a stepchild of medicine—virtually since its discovery in 1922? The pro and contra camps are clearly and vigorously, often violently, divided. The objectives of this book are to make available to the reader certain information on vitamin E which has appeared in the scientific literature since about 1960 and to assess what these publications say. Only very few of the articles that appeared in medical publications before 1960 are discussed here. Not that 1960 is a magic figure in the life of vitamin E, but a figure that is comparatively recent; by 1960 the variety of claims for vitamin E had somewhat settled down. People feel strongly about vitamin E and either praise it unduly or duly damn it. Both cannot be right. My own feeling is that both are wrong; but we do need an assessment without passion—especially because vitamin E does not do a thing in another passion, i.e., impotence, which was at one time but not anymore claimed for it.

This book is not sponsored by any manufacturer or distributor of vitamin E. It is not intended as an aid to the sale of vitamin E.

Attention is also directed to the fact that if this book is displayed with or otherwise assembled in conjunction with a vitamin E product in store windows or counters, it may well be considered to be advertising for such products; thus such display would be in violation of the Federal Food, Drug and Cosmetic Act. This point is especially called to the attention of health food or other stores that carry books in conjunction with the sale of food supplements.

Some aspects of vitamin E's functions, such as the relationship between polyunsaturated fatty acids and vitamin E, are explained in more than one chapter but in different contexts. This allows you to read the chapters consecutively without the need to refer again to previous chapters. In fact, I organized the book in a manner that would offer the clearest picture if the pages are read consecutively.

E. D.

CHAPTER 1

What Is Vitamin E?

King George III had it and lost the American colonies with his shenanigans. He had porphyria.

While people do not lose American colonies regularly, they can have other troubles if they have porphyria. They can get abdominal pain that is frequently severe enough to be like a colic, with vomiting and diarrhea, or they can develop psychiatric problems with delusions and hallucinations (such are said to have been King George III's problems, and only recently has it been decided that they were due to porphyria). Or porphyria can affect breathing and cause paralysis of respiration; or it can increase pigmentation of the skin, especially when exposed to light; or it can particularly cause a wide distribution of blisters on the skin.

The cause of porphyria is genetic. The disease occurs when nature slips a cog, when it does not give the individual affected the ability to produce a certain enzyme. The missing enzyme differs with the several kinds of porphyria. But in all of them there is one common abnormality: porphyrins and similar pigments are overproduced and accumulate in different organs, as well as in the blood, depending on the kind of porphyria. They are also excreted in the urine, but enough, too much, remain in the body to create havoc. Normally, the urine contains only traces.

Porphyria itself is a rare enough condition—and there are several kinds of porphyria, each kind affecting different organs. Although rare, when a person gets it, it is 100% when it hits him. Heretofore, a variety of drugs were used without success, that is, until the stepchild of therapeutics, vitamin E, was tried.

Dr. P. P. Nair, director of the biochemistry research division of the department of medicine of the Sinai Hospital of Baltimore, and his associates, Drs. Mezey, Quartner, and Murti, are credited with that discovery. In fact, a paper, published in the September 1971 issue of the highly respected *Archives of Internal Medicine,* gives details on several cases and discusses vitamin E and porphyrin metabolism in man.

But you will not be faced with treating your porphyria. As a matter of fact you cannot treat it yourself. This brief account of porphyria is given to broaden the view of what areas and corners vitamin E finds a place. And while it does not succeed in some areas it finds a place in others.

Vitamin E in animals and man.

Vitamin E is a fascinating and often paradoxical vitamin. Although it is a vitamin in which dramatic deficiency signs, such as those of scurvy in vitamin C deficiency, are not known, it is probably found in a greater number of body tissues than any other vitamin. Other vitamin deficiencies show their effect in the malfunction of one or a few body systems; but a chronic deficiency of vitamin E can affect *all* body systems in animals and *many* body systems in man.

For example, in animals, vitamin E deficiency can

manifest itself in various symptoms in different tissues, such as: in rats and fowl, a deficiency causes inability to reproduce; in dogs, lambs, rabbits, chicks, pigs, and monkeys, deficiency can produce a disease of muscles (muscular dystrophy) which can immobilize the animal; in monkeys, deficiency can produce anemia; in chicks too little vitamin E can cause nerve degeneration (encephalomalacia); in pigs a deficiency can bring about disease of the muscles of motion as well as of the heart muscle; in many other animals vitamin E deficiency can produce degeneration of the kidney or liver and the formation of a curious pigment called ceroid, which often accompanies certain degenerative processes.

Consistent with the broad role that vitamin E apparently has, its use in man has been described throughout the world medical literature in the treatment of various conditions, including: heart disease; other circulatory dysfunctions, such as peripheral vascular disease in which circulation is impeded (one such is intermittent claudication) or in which clots form in the veins in the leg (thrombophlebitis); symptoms of the menopause; burns, in which it is used both internally and externally; dysfunction of fat metabolism (malabsorption syndrome); and some of the respiratory effects of pollution. More recently, vitamin E's use in preventing or reversing certain anemias caused by the destruction of blood cells (hemolysis) in newborn or premature babies has received authoritative and serious consideration.

Frank deficiency of vitamin E—with classic deficiency symptoms—is not known in man except in certain anemias of premature infants and in malabsorption. That is not a blessing but a severe drawback. It has contributed to complicating the role of vitamin E. But serious research is going on. One example is the serious and painstaking reports on the mechanism and role of vitamin E—the subject of the International Conference on Vitamin E sponsored by the New York Academy of

Sciences held in December 1971 in New York. A section at the end of this book reports on the papers read at the Symposium.

Succeeding chapters of this book will describe important conditions in which the use of vitamin E has been reported and in which it can be useful. Chapters are devoted to more recent reports on the use of vitamin E in aging that, although no clear evidence exists, may well bear consideration. Surely, serious and diligent investigations are merited in order to determine the role of vitamin E in health and disease since the chances are high that it will pay good dividends. In fact, in research, it is just as important to determine that a given substance is not useful in a given condition, as it is to determine that it is useful.

The resistance against vitamin E is not really extraordinary when we recall that James Lind, a Scottish physician, published his "Treatise on the Scurvy" in 1753, and proved that lime juice prevents and cures it. Yet, despite the fact that the death rate for sailors from scurvy was unusually high, it was more than 40 years before the British Navy supplied sailors with daily lime juice rations as an absolute preventative of scurvy.

It is almost expected that a substance which is reputed to be useful for everything will be considered to be useful for nothing. During the 1940s and 1950s vitamin E went into a period of eclipse during which it was offered without foundation—a matter of commercial exploitation—for a variety of conditions. Perhaps that is one reason why vitamin E was so long a stepchild of medicine.

The tocopherols.

Vitamin E is one of the fat-soluble vitamins—like vitamins A, D, and K. Yet, in a number of functional respects it is similar to vitamin C, which is a water-soluble vitamin. For example, the highest concentration of vitamin E, like vitamin C, is found in the adrenals; vitamin E is a natural antioxidant like vitamin C; and it resembles vitamin C in other respects too. In fact there may be a metabolic relationship between vitamin E and vitamin C because in certain animals vitamin E is necessary for the synthesis of vitamin C.

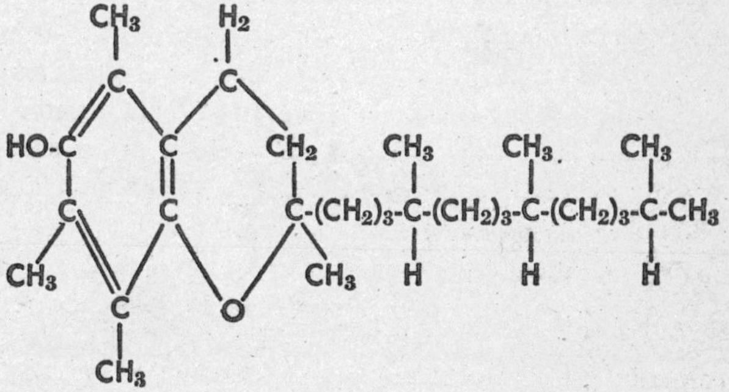

```
       CH3     H2
        |      |
        C      C
      //  \  /   \
  HO-C     C      CH2     CH3        CH3        CH3
     |     ||      |       |          |          |
     C     C       C-(CH2)3-C-(CH2)3-C-(CH2)3-C-CH3
    /  \\ /  \   /  \       |          |          |
 CH3    C     O      CH3    H          H          H
        |
       CH3
```

alpha-tocopherol

Vitamin E is also known by its chemical name, tocopherol. But not all tocopherols or vitamins E are the same. There are variants of vitamin E—the variants are called isomers—which, although chemically identical, differ in their biological potency. These principal isomers are called alpha-, beta-, gamma-, and delta-tocopherols—expressed as α-, β-, γ-, and δ- tocopherols. (There are also minor variants of tocopherol with fractional activity—such as epsilon-tocopherol, zeta-tocopherol, and eta-tocopherol—which have no vitamin E activity.)

Alpha-tocopherol (α-tocopherol) is the most active biologically.

Here is a rundown of the relative potencies of the alpha-tocopherols:

Vitamin E Activity of 1 mg. of Various Tocopherols

	International Units per 1 mg.
dl-alpha-tocopheryl acetate	1.
dl-alpha-tocopherol	1.1
d-alpha-tocopheryl acetate	1.36
d-alpha-tocopherol	1.49
d-alpha-tocopheryl succinate	1.21

Compare with other than the alpha isomers:

d-beta-tocopherol	0.4
d-gamma-tocopherol	0.2
dl-gamma-tocopherol	0.15
d-delta-tocopherol	0.016
dl-delta-tocopherol	0.012

The α-tocopheryl acetate or succinate, which are called esters, are derivatives of alpha-tocopherol, while tocopherol is chemically designated an alcohol. The alcohol is called a tocopher*ol* (all alcohols end in *ol*); an ester is called tocopher*yl* (the *yl* ending is that of an ester). Esters are chemical compounds of an alcohol and an acid; thus the tocopheryl esters available for use in man, as tablets or capsules, are the acetate and succinate esters—compounds of tocopherol with acetic and succinic acid respectively.

The reason that the esters are used is based on the experience that the esterified form (acetate or succinate) is more resistant to oxidation or other spoilage. The physiologic effects are the same. In fact the international standard is an ester, *dl*-α-tocopherol acetate, of which 1 milligram (mg.) is equivalent to 1 International Unit (I.U.).

What about the *d*, the *l* and the *dl* forms of vitamin E? They stand for *dextro, levo*, and for *dextro-levo* respectively. (The *d* and *l* forms are chemically identical but on physical tests show a difference in how they rotate a beam of light.) In many other materials there are often considerable differences in potencies between *d* and *l* forms. With vitamin E, or α-tocopherol, both the *d* and *l* forms are active—with a higher activity for the *d* form. But that is not of consequence because the amount used of either form is easily adjusted to give the number of International Units desired. However, the reason that the *dl* mixture is preferably used in vitamin E preparations is based on the finding that the *dl* form (called a racemic mixture), although not necessarily more active, is better absorbed when administered than if either the *d* or *l* form were given separately.

This is a phenomenon of considerable importance in the administration of almost any drug. A small difference in a chemical or drug may have profound differences in absorption in the body. If there is no absorption, there is no utilization of the body (except for drugs that act locally, such as in coating a tissue). In other words, biological activity rather than chemical configuration is the determining factor in the utilization of most substances.

Absorption also has another factor, the inability of an individual to absorb fats. This is discussed in the chapter on malabsorption. In addition, there are also individual differences in the constitution of people that often control absorption.

Natural versus synthetic.

There are two kinds of vitamin E available: the natural and synthetic. The natural is made by distillation of vegetable oils under vacuum or by extraction of vegetable oils by solvents. The synthetic is chemically produced. But both are identical in effect—each is tested biologically to assure that the effect is physiologically the same. The natural form, weight for weight, is stronger in vitamin E activity, but that is of no actual consequence because all vitamin E products are adjusted to contain a given amount of vitamin E activity in terms of International Units, and are sold *in terms of International Units.*

The dispute between the virtues of natural versus synthetic materials is still alive. When the chemical nature of a substance is known—as with vitamin E—there is no difference between the natural and synthetic forms, assuming that the strengths are biologically tested. As an example, vitamins B_1, C, D, as well as E—whether from natural or synthetic sources—are identically the same. In fact, the goodness of the natural variety is tested against the pure synthetic material to see if it, the natural, conforms to the standard, which is synthetic. Much if not most of the dispute between those who prefer natural over synthetic origins is often, but not always, based on emotional or commercial considerations. The naturally derived variety of most substances costs more. This is not an attack against materials of natural origin; it cannot be, for we take the position that there is no difference in a well-defined chemical substance between natural and synthetic origin.

But there are exceptions. For example, a naturally derived vitamin B complex may possibly have advantages as it may contain yet undiscovered or not yet chemically characterized components of the vitamin B complex. But in clearly characterized components of the vitamin B complex, such as thiamine or vitamin B_1, there is no difference.

In other cases a synthetically derived vitamin may be superior. For example, orange juice contains vitamin C of natural origin. But if an infant is sensitive or allergic to orange juice, the administration of vitamin C tablets (in which the vitamin C is synthetically derived) is vastly superior. The reason is that orange juice contains, in addition to vitamin C, substances to which the infant is sensitive.

Returning to vitamin E: unless the material from natural sources is biologically tested, it may contain isomers of vitamin E which are not biologically active. A chemical test alone does not distinguish among the isomers, as the answer given in a chemical test shows only the total amount of tocopherols in a given sample.

Destroyers of vitamin E.

Vitamin E is often found in multivitamin tablets and capsules which contain other vitamins and minerals. A fair though not a sufficient amount of vitamin E is found in these mixtures. But a serious drawback resides in depending on vitamin E from multivitamin-mineral combinations if such combinations contain iron. Although there is a need for iron in daily nutrition and it may be wiser to take it than to depend on obtaining enough iron from food, iron and vitamin E are not compatible. The amount of vitamin E in such multivitamin-mineral preparations is functionally not useful, as it is destroyed by taking it with iron.

But multivitamin-mineral preparations as well as vitamin E can be taken daily, provided that one is taken in the morning and the other one in the evening.

In succeeding chapters reference is made to polyunsaturated fatty acids—in which vegetable oils are rich—and how they also detrimentally affect the vitamin E intake in man.

Toxicity.

Vitamin E has one outstanding feature in that toxic effects are not known in man. This aspect of vitamin E has been tested by many investigators, and no untoward effect has been reported. The only note of caution was sounded by Dr. Evan V. Shute, who believes that vitamin E should be given with care in rheumatic heart disease, as its effect in strengthening the contractions of the heart is so rapid that considerable harm may result, unless administered only in small and gradually increasing doses. Dr. Shute has been in the vanguard of vitamin E investigation. Although his reports were once considered overoptimistic, glowing results with vitamin E have also been reported by investigators from many other parts of the world.

Vitamin E has had its detractors, and in some cases they may well have been justified. But it is easier and safer to be negative than to put one's name and reputation on the line—which requires courage. For that reason perhaps, many detractors hold on to their negative approach, rather than take on a searching attitude. To quote Lancelot Hogben:

> A scientific hypothesis must live dangerously or die of inanition. Science thrives on daring generalizations. There is nothing particularly scientific about excessive caution. Cautious explorers do not cross the Atlantic of truth.*

* "Science for the Citizen," *Science*, Oct. 8, 1954, p. 582.

CHAPTER 2

What Does "Aging" Mean?

The role of vitamin E is only one aspect of aging, though an important one if the antioxidant theory is largely correct. Other facets of aging include the social and behavioral, the general state of natural resistance and health, the emotional and mental, financial, occupational and recreational, spiritual, and nutritional ones. Nor are these conditions listed in an order of importance—they vary in importance with each person. For example, a person in good physical health who is slowly dying of boredom in his retirement will find that the emotional aspect (where he is a factor in the constellation of his family) is more important than his physical health—if you actually can separate physical from emotional health. Or, a person ostensibly in excellent physical and emotional state will find the financial aspects of aging to be of paramount concern if he is forced to live on the dole that social security pays him, to keep him on just this side of starvation.

While aging is a deadly disease, it need not at all be a step contiguous to the exit. And unlike other diseases —if you think of age in terms of disease—you do not want to eliminate it: the only way to a long life is through aging. Nor do you want to get off the boat, because you may well soon reach a new plateau, replete with satisfactions, while aging. This may well occur if you examine life during and especially *before* aging dispassionately and thoughtfully and make changes which can make age a pleasant stage. We make continuous changes when we go from adolescence into maturity. Change is the staff of life.

Change is unpleasant for many people—until they effect the necessary change. Charles Kettering (1876-1958), one of the outstanding inventive minds of this century whose basic inventions made automobile pollution possible, had a marvelous comment on this subject: "If you have always done it that way it is probably wrong."

Age—a state of mind.

Aging is a gradual process, but above all, it is a *state of mind*. Aging does not mean being in the 80s or 70s necessarily—for it increasingly applies to all of us. It applies to a person in the 40s, for in fact, he is relatively more aged than he was in his 30s. If you feel that you are old today, take courage: a year hence you will look back at having been a year younger and will regret that you did not enjoy or experience certain sensations which you thought then you were too old to undertake, or at least in which to participate.

Only nincompoops make youth a career itself. Perhaps Winston Churchill's (1874–1965) comment that the young sow wild oats and the old grow sage (hopefully) may be well applied here. While age and maturity are not necessarily the same, wisdom is one of the dividends we can draw from age, hopefully. None of us know we are young until we have passed it. For example, a man or woman in the 50s does not consider himself or herself young—but 10 years later will look back to the 50s as the time of having been young or younger.

If you say that age is a state of years, not a state of mind, you will be partially correct. But functionally, what you do and how you feel during any period is what makes the conduct of your life or your enjoyment of it. We do not live in terms of years but in terms of our activities. And our activities are based on what our self-image is at a given time, the mental or emotional cast in which we view ourselves.

Perhaps one test of age—and there are many—and of our mental and emotional view of ourselves is whether we look back or look ahead. Offhand this may appear to be an oversimplification, but actually it is not. For example, an aged person whose only contact with his contemporaries consists of reminiscences is looking back, and he virtually cuts off his view of his future. He makes no plans because he sees no future, and it becomes a self-fulfilling prophecy: his dwelling on the past is cutting off his future. His horizon contracts and his interest in events external to him shrinks.

Learning and experience.

One of the activities which suggests youth rather than aging is the ability to learn. This is not meant in terms of structured, formal instruction—though that also applies—but the ability to make a change in the accustomed way we have continued to do things, presumably, so successfully. For example, if you find that your young new neighbor cannot really teach you anything new about, say, how to make fried eggs—because you have been doing it for 40 years—you are aging, but fast.

And wouldn't you be horrified if a young person tells you how you can better enjoy a sexual encounter—you, who have had all that experience for all those years?

Experience should not necessarily be denigrated—

but experience often means that you may have had a long history of doing a thing in less than an optimal fashion.

The willingness and ability to try a new insight or a new approach is the ability to learn. One of the outstanding hallmarks of being young in mind is the ability or the courage to learn.

Negativeness.

Another trait concomitant with aging is negativeness —holding a foregone conclusion that "it will not work," without having the probative experience to that effect. People fear to fail—as if the failure of an experiment reflects upon their person. A hallmark of youth is when you *fail to fear rather than fear to fail.* Youth—not in years but in mind—has an affirmative cast. It will not discard an idea unless it has experimentally determined that it does not work. Many of the great innovators—young or old in years though all were young as to their state of mind—found that when an experiment in something new had failed the design of the experiment was at fault, not necessarily the idea. For example, the expression "606" is well known—it refers to the "magic bullet," the first time successful chemotherapy of syphilis was discovered by Paul Ehrlich (1854-1915). The reason it was called 606 is because 605 experiments failed—the 606th one succeeded. (When we view the rising incidence of syphilis in the latter half of the 20th century, perhaps he should not have stopped at the 606th experiment. Surely, he did not run out of syphilis spirochetes.)

A negative trait is akin to cynicism, just as cynicism is an accentuation of a negative side of endeavors. If you take an attitude of cynicism it is like saying that nothing works and even if it does it is an accident; which merely shows that you can't even trust your foregone conclusion that nothing works. The damage that cynicism produces is, unfortunately, largely to the cynic. If nothing is expected to result to the good, nothing does.

Another characteristic of aging is that we take natural phenomena for granted. When you stop wondering at the enormity of creation—from the effect of an insignificant enzyme to the whole constitution of what makes man—you have aged. A child continues to wonder—and thereby grows emotionally, as well as physically.

Accentuation of existing traits.

In aging, we find that traits predominant during our younger days become accentuated. Regrettably, this applies more particularly to the negative, the undesirable traits. For example, when a person during his adult years is given to being suspicious, that trait sometimes becomes exaggerated to the point of caricature as the years progress. He may extend suspiciousness over a larger area of daily events or view new things with more intense suspicion. Such a situation may progress until his trait becomes more properly a paranoid way of thinking—with its delusions of persecution when an untoward event precipitates an alarm reaction.

But we must be wary of calling our own traits the prudence of skepticism and those in others as cynicism or paranoia. It gives us a feeling of comfort—by reducing our own ambiguities and anxieties—to project on others traits which we would not like to believe to be true to us. But it does no constructive good to others or ourselves.

If age is a state of mind, it appears to be wisdom to act in consistency with the "young" state of mind. For example, New York City occasionally gives evidence of its municipal wisdom; one such step is to offer half-fare privileges on its miserable transportation to people who show a senior citizen card. Many men and women do not avail themselves of that crumb from the festive table of municipal corruption, because it would make them *feel* old. They pay full inflated fare rather than reduce the strength of the image of how they look upon themselves—a logical and wise move.

While the difference between full and half fare is not payment to a guaranteed state of mind, it is a wise move. Even a small step adds or detracts from the total image. A posture people assume has many components. But despite the label of "senior citizen," no one has been reported thus far as considering surrender of citizenship to get out of the class label. Senior alien may be worse.

Longevity.

The practical aspects in increasing the life span—assuming it will happen as prognosticated by the prophets or wishful thinkers of science—will create problems which from this vantage point are horrendous. Imagine an increase from the average of 70 years to a common event of death at 90. Questions immediately suggested are: Would that be a lengthening of the misery of the old? Will that be merely an accentuation of senility which will endure longer? Or, will man be vigorous until the day he dies—whether at 70 or 90?

Whatever the scientific advances have in store, one point is inescapable: an increase in lifespan without an increase in content and substance would be at best meaningless, and at worse a grave disservice. It would be equivalent to converting prisons into luxurious hotels but lengthening the sentences. Such luxury without the freedom outside of prison would probably be sought by very few, unless we convert our prisons to a co-ed basis. But we have a paucity of women convicts to make it workable.

Thus, perhaps the wisest objective now is to improve the *content* of life in the later years, even though the lifespan is not yet increased. The fortunate point is that such an enrichment of content is available now, to every individual, provided that he or she is aware of the ingredients that improve such content. Most people know that barring existing, or developing disease, the emotional content is what enriches life, and conversely, the greatest destructive force in life is boredom. What can be done toward those aims? There are now about 20 million people in the United States 65 years old and older. Their number is increasing—a population explosion that contraceptives, oral or any other kind, cannot cure.

Health.

There is immense activity coupled with agitation to conquer cancer. But if we stop to assess these fine aspirations we become somewhat disquieted: statisticians find that while the conquest of cancer will add years to older people, it will add only 1½ years on the whole to our life expectancy at 65. People will continue to die from degenerative diseases—and less strikingly but more slowly of boredom.

Perhaps we should adjust our prejudices: it does not matter much from what we die (cancer, etc.) as long as we are able to live reasonably joyously, not merely comfortably, within the existing lifespan. The realistic objective is a vigorous span of the later years and not merely postponement of the cause of death.

Such a view of the population at large is hardly a comfort to those with cancer. But we should at least define our viewpoint.

A comforting thought comes from the noted British geriatrician happily named Alex Comfort, director of Medical Research of the Council Group on Biology of

Aging, at the University College, London, who believes that by 1990 vigorous life will be prolonged by 20 years.

If you have parents, you may wonder what problems the increase of life will accentuate. The candid facts are that many people consider their parents a cross to bear. The more affluent expiate their hostile feeling by boarding their parents at nursing homes—a step from the grave. It would be constructive to project ourselves 20 or 25 years hence when we will have reached the same age. It is only then that we can truly assess the value of a longer life without content or substance.

How will life be lengthened? Partially by application of research results yet to come—and partially by application now, of what we know.

Sleep and food.

In addition to treatment for diseases which exhibit symptoms, and periodic surveillance by a physician, an individual can do much in his day-by-day endeavors to heighten his physical well-being.

One of them is sleep. The myths agree that older people need less sleep—and perhaps the myths persist because older people rise much earlier than the customary hour of 7 A.M. which is considered "normal." But upon reflection we find that older people do not necessarily awaken earlier because they cannot sleep. One of the reasons they awaken so much earlier is because they retire earlier and thus get an approximation of their hitherto normal amount of sleep. Another reason for their early morning awakening is depression —due largely and probably to their lowering of self-esteem and feeling of usefulness, the feeling of loneliness accentuated by the increasingly frequent loss of friends and older family members and the resulting anxieties such losses engender. It all adds up to—

boredom the most fertile soil for behavioral anomalies.

But recent work has confirmed the view that older people need as much sleep as other adults. If anything, they may need more sleep due to its reparative function.

Another myth is that older people need less food. They do need a better balance, which may total less in quantity—only the type differs. They need more protein due to its reconstructive function, less fat and carbohydrates, and more of the accessory food elements, such as vitamins and minerals. The reason why more protein is necessary—barring individual or genetic needs—is because repair of tissue is not as efficient as in the younger adults. For that reason, anabolic steroid injections are often recommended for older people. Anabolic steroids are similar to testosterone—although this also has an anabolic effect. Anabolism is construction of tissue or muscle mass. These agents help the building of protein and conserve its loss.

Calcium is needed because of the prevalence of osteoporosis as age increases. Osteoporosis is thinning of bone by loss of calcium. This is not the whole story because it is also related to the utilization of calcium which requires vitamin D and to other hormonal influences.

Nutrition.

An adequate vitamin intake is highly desirable. The principal reason is that the utilization of vitamins is less efficient in older than in younger people; another reason is that it helps stimulate the function of the enzymes, which are necessary in most functions of the body. Perhaps a major reason is due to the fact that personal eccentricity in food habits may not allow an adequate intake of the variety of accessory food elements that are optimum to good nutrition.

There are many reports that the lack of mental acuity and even confused mental states considered to be due to senility have been remedied by a high vitamin intake. Whether that is due to the effect of the vitamins per se, or whether a subclinical vitamin deficiency was present, is not known. A high vitamin intake is especially needed by people in their 70s or older, particularly those in a low economic level whose food intake is largely toast, jam, potatoes, and tea. It may well be true in a less dramatic measure in others. Senility is a comfortable diagnosis for the one who makes it—it discharges the need for thoughtful and compassionate attention. But senility reversed is a thrill to attain.

The need for calories decreases with age, but food intake should not be curtailed at the expense of proteins. The reason for the lower caloric need is based on the lower energy needs, lessened activity, and the lower metabolic rate, which means less energy expenditure. In addition, overeating has a role in increasing the incidence and severity of degenerative diseases, such as heart and kidney dysfunctions.

While overeating is a problem with older people, existing obesity is probably not as threatening as with younger people. The former did reach the age they are at, despite obesity. While obesity is surely not recommended, drastic or even vigorous reducing regimens are probably more thoughtless ritual than wisdom. In order to have the advantage of a protein- and vitamin-rich food intake, dry skimmed milk and yeast can be an important part of the diet. A predinner cocktail prepared of dry skimmed milk with yeast and water in a blender may be used to "spoil the appetite" as a guard against overeating at dinner.

People often speak of a vegetarian diet as an ideal diet and proudly point to George Bernard Shaw as an exponent. They forget a few pertinent factors: Hitler was also a vegetarian, and each delivered deadly barbs —Shaw verbally and Hitler militaristically. Is there a relationship here, which suggests any inherent cannibalism as a substitute for a meat diet?

Another rationalization for a vegetarian diet is the evidence that certain African tribes who eat no meat do not develop heart disease and arteriosclerosis or cancer. True. The examples thus far are based on fact and are evidence of the logical application of a concept.

But remind your meatless evangelists that there are other African tribes that exist solely on a meat, blood, and milk diet who also are not known to develop heart disease, arteriosclerosis, or cancer—all of which are ascribed to a meat diet by meatless evangelists.

Increasing age is a time when the individual frenetically seeks for some method of arresting its progress. Little does a person realize that the only absolute way to arrest age is by death. In this energetic search for eternal youth he often embraces fads. It is true that the fads of one era at times become the accepted dogma 30 or 40 years later. But that is not generally true. Though fads are not frequently harmful, they pose certain hazards. Some (such as meatless diets) may be hazards when they militate against good nutrition. Others are inadvisable since they waste time—you can be following a desirable regimen rather than putting your energy into fads.

It is often difficult to determine what is, or will turn out to be, a fad. Brewer's yeast started as a fad and rose—no pun intended—to the position of an acceptable food substance.

Yoga exercises began as a fad. If one remains open-minded, one must conclude that they have a salutory effect. Part of it may be due to the physical exercise and part to the reduction of tension induced by contemplation. It does not matter if the effect is that of a placebo—which we doubt that it is—but if it offers weight reduction, a method of exercise, and tension release, it is all to the good.

Placebos too have their effect to the good if your aim is individual well-being. Hope, to the extent that it reduces tension and increases emotional well-being, also is positive and wholesome.

Emotional.

Any separation between physical and emotional well-being is faulty, or at best only one-sided. And the one side is incomplete. Paradoxically, it is simpler to get attention for the physical components of well-being—especially if they are severe—than to the emotional. In the emotional area of daily living, the factors leading to sound practices are strangely enough more easily implemented by the individual himself. How? Through the understanding of the needs and factors involved. This does not mean that psychotherapy is useless or unnecessary. The question is where and when to use it. Surely, many of the common dissatisfactions arising from boredom can escalate over a period of time and require psychotherapy. But many of the problems of daily living can be largely ameliorated by looking into probable causes and applying proposed remedies.

For example, the retired person who had not planned for retirement can find activities that are more than occupational therapy, can yet raise his self-esteem and therewith give some meaning to life. You don't ask a psychotherapist what to do when you are bored. The resourcefulness of searching yourself increases your own resourcefulness.

Children who are on vacation, freed from school duties, often approach their mothers with the plea: "What shall I play now?" They get bored with the sameness. Older people who lack substantial resourcefulness often are in the same position.

This is acutely borne out by the example of a union that negotiates a four-day week. Many workers find time hanging on their hands and take a moonlighting job, or worse, spend time in a bar to kill the extra time. They have not yet learned how to convert leisure time into an enriching experience.

Whole well-being depends largely on emotional well-being—composed of self-fulfillment, self-esteem, and a reasonably interesting activity.

Self-esteem.

If you have parents, whether living in your household or not, you feel a responsibility, an attachment, or even a hostility to them. How to *handle* them is often a problem. But the fault is not with the aged, according to Dr. Ewald W. Busse, president of the American Psychiatric Association, as recounted in the *Psychiatric Reporter* of April 21, 1971. Busse considers the aged a "deprived minority" and most of their problems to arise from loss of self-esteem. Even though biologic changes are concomitant with age, the sociologic changes, he avers, focus the problems to an acuteness that is destructive to the aged: "Society fails to provide recreational and educational opportunities that are essential to maintaining self-esteem and acceptable activity levels in old age."

Superficially, Busse can be refuted by mentioning that senior citizens' group camps are offered to the elderly. But such "golden age clubs" are virtually concentration camps with free access and departure. Society does not make provisions for preventing disuse of the faculties of the aged in a work relationship—and such a policy eventually results in atrophy.

"An individual must feel he is valued or appreciated by others in order to have a reasonable esteem of his own self," according to Dr. Busse; most societally oriented scientists will concur.

The importance of self-esteem was realized even by

the ancients, to whom human feelings were not commonly of concern. Caecilius Statius (220–167 B.C.), stated: "People can bear hardship easily as long as there is no injury, and yet they can bear injury without much difficulty as long as they do not need to cope with insult."

We may well concede that the aged are the truly underprivileged, or deprived, minority. Most of the 20 million of them are in the lower and middle socioeconomic levels. Those in the higher socioeconomic levels are less affected by this discrimination, because the events of aging *are* related to the environment—whether the environment is familial, societal, or economic. It would thus be expected, and it does follow, that those people who are on a higher level through education or occupation during their prime of life commonly retain intelligence and a *show of youth* probably longer than those not so privileged. In this aspect too, Dr. Busse concurs; his position is that the gradual loss of brain cells alone, which occurs daily from the prime of life onwards, does not seem to be an adequate explanation for the impairment of memory and intellect with advancing years.

The show of youth.

But should all be blamed on the environment? Far from it. All of us are partially architects of our own decline: we virtually signal the rate of decline by our own actions or by failing to take certain actions.

Decline is inexorable. What is of preeminent concern is the *rate* at which it proceeds. Much as with money: obviously, if we spend our resources to buy inconsequential baubles, soon we will not have enough resources left to buy something of outstanding value—even at bargain prices. In other words, the rate of outflow has been too great to sustain our resources.

Sudden aging is a rare thing. It can come after a cataclysmic and sudden event upon which the individual exposed to it suddenly feels old—and therefore becomes old. But that is rare. Aging is a gradual process, and how fast it occurs is a matter of rate. In fact, rate figures in most of our activities. That is the reason why, in the poor state of our knowledge, we should take advantage of what we know about aging. And there is little dissent from the view that anything we can do to retard the rate of aging is positive and sound.

One common quality found in individuals to whom the approach to advancing years is a burden is that virtually all of them lack an interest. This is a lack of interest in *some* activity (not necessarily a hobby)—a lack of interest in people, or in the world around them, or in their own committal to something.

The interest must be a viable thing, a strong concern, not merely a meek and mild show of things. At its best, it is a passionate involvement. It is wisely deduced—and has been confirmed—that people with many interests are least exposed to or suffer least from boredom, the king of the men of death for those approaching or who have attained agedness.

Interest is not something that an individual pursues because it's "good for him," such as exercise, which is a different matter. It is an activity for which his soul hungers. It does not matter if the interest is in counting the number of steps going up—to check if it is the same number going down. Interest need not be in the arts per se—although if a person is fortunate enough to have a sincere involvement in one of the arts he has truly a creative interest. Nor should what the neighbors think be of concern. What's wrong with collecting books which have 269 pages—no more, no less—if that satisfies an urge, even if it is eccentric?

Don't let the word "eccentric" frighten you. It means merely *out of the center*. In that way it is an interest which is out of the center, out of the average. It may set you off from the average, and though to your face people may laugh tolerantly, secretly they may admire an eccentric interest and admire the man or woman who has the courage to follow his interest. The British are known for their eccentricities—is that one reason why they wrinkle much later than Americans?

But eccentricity must be judged by some standard of good sense. A man of 75 who had an interest in collecting dog excrement of various colors should probably have thought in advance that at least a matter of public health was involved.

The discussion of the variety of interests requires volumes; their evaluation many more. But we can draw from them one important point, namely, that a viable interest is one in which the individual is *active*. Interest, like democracy, is not a spectator sport.

More specifically, an interest in viewing TV is not an interest that is viable in the sense of this discussion—at best it is a vicarious enterprise, which substitutes passivity for activity. A viable interest is an active thing; it includes collecting, producing, evaluating, choosing—all active components. Being a recipient—a brainwashed vessel into which ideas are allowed to fall—is not a viable activity which enhances emotional equilibrium. People are happiest when they are contributing—in their rest periods or between them.

A strong involvement in an interest usually leads to a creative attitude. Creativeness is basically present in every individual. During our working years it is often suppressed because industry and the economic world roll on the tracks of mediocrity. A creative person often rocks the boat—though in the final analysis he can confer enduring benefits to society.

But interest and creativeness do not suddenly make their appearance at 65—the magic but irrational number that signals retirement. They are lifelong devotions

—the respites that reduce the frustrations and disappointments that invariably are part of our working years. Hence, the choice and practice of an interest—*early in life*—assures a building up of inner resources which bar boredom and enhance emotional equilibrium. Age is a state of mind, not a sum of years. Hence interest and creativeness lessen the rate of aging, assuming of course that no primary physical problems of age intervene.

Creativeness, too, is a state of mind and not necessarily a masterpiece of painting or music or literature. A masterpiece is merely a manifestation of creativeness. Do not measure the goodness of your interest by what artistic or creative manifestations it produces. The test is your emotional involvement in your interest. Creativeness takes many forms.

Depression.

Aging is a matter of deterioration—gradual but inexorable. All structures and senses deteriorate, but fortunately *the mind is usually the last to deteriorate,* provided that emotional and environmental support are received and that interest in the environment is retained. (This is one reason why people at a higher socioeconomic level age much more slowly. Owing to earlier education and activities, they have a greater involvement with their environment and retain their interest. Another reason is nutritional.) With a loss of interest something else takes its place: depression.

Depression associated with aging is largely the result of boredom, a lack of interest in the environment—with nothing to take its place. Few things take place in a vacuum—nature fills its vacuums; and it is our privilege to choose with what our personal vacuum is to be filled. We can develop or choose an interest and remain active in it—or else nature sends depression to fill the empty space.

This does not mean that depression, especially among those in the prime of life or in the young, always has the same pattern, cause, and remedy. Depression may be a serious state requiring psychopharmacologic intervention. We are talking only of the depression arising from lack of interest (hence boredom) frequently seen in those past the prime of life, in those whose emotional resources have not been nurtured during their youth and their prime. In such people depression is the alternative that fills the empty tracks of living. And deterioration goes on at a faster rate in the presence of such depression connected with aging. Hence, aging is accelerated.

Depression hastily brings other undesirable phenomena which accentuates aging—increases the rate of aging. Depression is tantamount to pessimism. Although pessimism logically follows repeated disappointments in financial, familial, occupational, and other matters, the dangers of pessimism are formidable when they become a way of life, a pattern, a life-style by which future events are measured. Pessimism too, may act as a self-fulfilling prophecy, as when we look with a foreboding of gloom upon a new prospective event that does not yet merit the pessimistic outlook. It deepens depression.

Other traits that depression produces are irascibility—which can turn off an otherwise glowing prospect. Impatience can militate against a growing interpersonal encounter—which can be an enduring good in approaching years. Forgetfulness will clearly be accentuated when irascibility and impatience combine to produce emotional turmoil, which fires forgetfulness to new and yet unexperienced heights. Moderate forgetfulness is often found during the prime of life and normally increases with age. But it is brought to a crescendo by the vicious cycle fueled by pessimism and depression. Yet, much can be done against that type of depression. Nurturing of an interest—a passionate involvement—is one remedy.

Sex.

One of the most frequent sequels of depression is impotence on the part of the male and lack of sex interest in the female. Our Puritan heritage willed us an ironic legacy—a cultural curse—namely, surreptitiousness about sex. Whatever the reason, people often consider the practice of sexual relations an unseemly act, not fit for people who have attained a certain age. The image of a retired husband who, approaching his wife amorously, is rebuffed by "act your age" is a potent poison to the practice of sexual endeavors. He is acting his age—without the Puritan myths which tell him how to act. But his wife has not yet examined the myth and probably wants to send her husband for another type of examination—a psychiatric one.

A highly prominent and active lawyer, widowed in his late 70s, who had long heard of the myth but never believed it, came to the attention of the public because his daughter, after a family quarrel, asked him at 2 A.M. to leave her house, which he was visiting in another city. It appears that the reason for the family argument was that the daughter, who believed the myth, objected to the fact that one of her father's mistresses was one of her own friends. Before that, another of her friends, living in the same city as her father, had also been a mistress of the lawyer. Further details were not available: the lawyer, because of his prominence, prevailed upon the judge before whom he was brought to hold the session in his chambers. The complaint was disturbing the peace—whereas the facts were that the daughter disturbed the father's peace. This incident is reminiscent of Oliver Wendell Holmes' wish: "Oh, to be 69 again."

The subject of sex has recently been more openly discussed and hence researched. There is a substantial agreement that sexual desire does not necessarily lessen with age—except in the case of depression. What is even more important is that by and large the ability to perform the sexual act does not markedly decline in the 50s, 60s, or even in the 70s. It becomes a self-fulfilling prophecy when the party line holds that a man should not "think of such things" at his age—when he is in his 50s or 60s.

The self-fulfilling prophecy becomes a reality through misinformation, according to Dr. James L. McCary, psychologist of the University of Houston, Texas. "And the tragedy is that misinformation not only becomes perpetuated by the distortions of truth communicated laterally by the peer group to its members, but also by those legitimately in a position to educate," he told a meeting at the Clinical Convention of the American Medical Association in Denver, in 1970. The myth about sexual desire and decreasing ability as persons age is just that—a myth.

Dr. McCary also reported that, according to his findings, about three-fourths (73%) of all men between the ages of 65 and 69 experience satisfactory coitus, as do about 60% of the men between the ages of 75 and 92. Further, his investigation disclosed that a consistent pattern of sexual intercourse during earlier years and at the prime helps retain sexual drive and ability into old age. But once interest is reduced, it is difficult to reestablish it.

These findings bear out the preeminent role of the mind (or more properly, the role of the emotions) upon the sex drive—a role which has long been well known—and also upon the ability to consummate sex relations, a theory which has only recently been widely accepted.

Impotence is largely a matter of the mind rather than of the body proper.

Since sex is one of the primary drives in life, it is an obvious conclusion that the loss of interest therein is a loss of the accouterments of youth—vigor, élan vital, and joy of living. Compare this with depression as a state of existence.

Unfortunately, when one speaks of sex and sex relations one too often speaks only of the role of and effect upon the male. What about the woman? It is deplorable indeed that much less attention is paid to the woman's needs and reactions and how they can be fructified.

One can simplify or oversimplify the relationship by stating that a man uses love to gain sex, while a woman uses sex to gain love.

In the childbearing age, the dynamics of man-woman relationships have their own unique constellation. But sex relations between adults past their childbearing and childrearing ages—when approaching old age—are something else again.

Partly because of biological and partly because of sociological reasons, a woman accommodates a man in his sex requirements. This does not mean that she does not have sex needs and aspirations—only that they are more delicately attuned and are not primarily based upon the need for release of tensions that the physical act performs for the man. Perhaps for that reason—and for other reasons—a woman's needs and satisfactions, are not as frequently considered as they should be.

Among woman's clear needs are concern, affection, and attention—in other words, the security of being a person in her own right, rather than just a necessary partner. Possibly because of our cultural and personal material values, no great effort is made by men to understand women's needs and to fulfill them. A man often acts as if in his financial care for her well-being he has discharged all his duties. Often he is all thumbs; that is, unless he puts his foot into the relationship.

A woman's need for empathy is present during all her life but is more particularly so as she approaches the menopause and after it. You cannot ask a woman to tell it in words. We have not developed our facility for nonverbal communication nearly as well as we have our straight black-and-white form of verbal communication. It is well to bear in mind that what is said verbally in an intimate relationship can be discounted 50% or possibly more. We say things more clearly and sincerely when our communication does not pass through the censor of our mind and is not expressed in subconsciously censored words. A woman often merely accommodates her husband or lover sexually, because the picture in her mind—of a widowed woman of her acquaintance or of one without a steady lover—lowers her socially, even in her own mind. She accommodates to raise the man's ego and often dissembles emotion in the act.

For example, a man noticed that in sexual congress, his mate always folded her arms across her chest. It was not her breasts that were cold but her attitude to her partner and the act. Instead of observing that this was a clear sign of her dissatisfaction with him or with the sex act, and determining how he could increase her satisfactions in life or otherwise, he complained that her elbows dug into his ribs. The fact that this happened repeatedly speaks for the denseness of both—or for the lack of honest communication between them. Surely, here was a severe disparity, which with attention and desire to please the other person probably could have been ameliorated.

A similar example where clear signs were ignored was when a woman always adroitly turned her face so that the man's kiss upon leaving always fell on her cheek. True, the man may have had bad breath and ugly teeth, but his real trouble was more likely emotional—mental rather than dental. He was dense in not looking further wherein the trouble lay.

These are some of the reasons why sex may be onerous to women—even though their need for sex exists. In fact, it is reported by one survey that about 30% of older married women supplement marital coitus with masturbation—which raises grand suspicions about the adequacy or wisdom of their husbands. Regrettably, men often do not give a damn after their orgasm.

The same survey has also found that of women who no longer have husbands 37% of those in their 50s and 12% of those in their 60s continue to have sex relationships. These matters suggest a reevaluation of our prejudices and cherished beliefs.

The practice of sex enhances the physical and emotional well-being of men and women during aging. This too suggests a rethinking of our man-woman relationships, emotionally and societally, and above all, a need for a realization on the part of men that an integral part of the sex act should be a concern for the emotional well-being of women.

When we speak of sex, we commonly refer to the usual heterosexual relationships. But we merely deplore the difficulties that the aging homosexual man or woman has in finding a satisfying sexual relationship. We should be looking at the problem with a view toward solution instead of sanctimoniously passing judgment.

The facts are that physically, as well as emotionally, the needs of homosexual men or women are the same as those of heterosexuals. Sex broadly is a drama in which the needs for power, dominance, surrender, affection, empathy, and finally self-esteem are needful to all human beings. Age is no bar—except for the barriers we *artificially* erect ourselves.

One of the few (thus far) stable observations is that

unless tremendous disparities exist, relationships in which there is mutually fulfilling sexual activity seldom fail. And the converse is also true. Yet, complaints of impotence are being reported at continuously earlier ages. A rethinking of our social values should be enlightening as to why this may be so.

Mind-body.

Our concern with the emotional aspects of aging frequently but erroneously is understood to be related only to our moods or our feelings. But its influence extends also to the physical parts of our well-being—a notion which has long been known.

There are many examples where emotional storms may have a profound role in purely physical events—if there is such a thing as the purely physical or the purely emotional. One report, from London's St. George's Hospital Medical School, by Dr. P. B. Storey, speaks of a study of 291 patients in whom stroke, with hemorrhage in the brain, was precipitated by emotional factors. Dr. Storey concludes from his experiences that emotional turmoil may be a more important diagnostic factor than angiograms in diagnosing the likelihood of the occurrence of stroke.

Another example is that given by Dr. J. H. Manhold, of the New Jersey College of Medicine and Dentistry. In a study recounting his experiments with rats, he found that social stress may well have a bearing on the development of disease of periodontal tissues. Persons in stressful situations responded with constriction of the blood vessels of the gums, hence the amount of oxygen coming to the tissues was restricted. They also showed other systemic symptoms, expectedly suggestive of a relative inhibition of the function of the adrenals (hypoadrenalism).

Age-accomplishment.

People often deny the existence of an unpleasant prospect—with the idle hope that it will go away by itself. Letting sleeping dogs lie, to use an awkward metaphor, is not a good policy because the dogs may not be asleep.

A wise approach appears to us to be an affirmative one. Admit that aging catches up with all of us—unless we die. But take what thoughtful steps you can in order to reduce its negative effects.

There are many faces to aging—and a variety of steps can be taken to ameliorate its bad effects or to postpone them by reducing the rate of approaching age. They have to do with the physical, spiritual, mental, occupational, and recreative ones, among others. One important attitude, in fact, in almost anything we do is committal. Committal, service to others, is not necessarily altruism. It may be merely intelligent selfishness in your interrelationships with your contemporaries, and it is another factor in emotional equilibrium. Compare that with the selfish, cantankerous stance ascribed to people as they age—and with their state of interactions with other people.

The objective of this chapter has been to discuss the emotional aspects of aging and how they can be assessed and converted to constructive ends. This is not a total picture—which would require volumes for a total explication.

We know too little about aging. But it would appear to be good judgment to utilize what we do know and what is largely accepted to be sound and salubrious. The attempt to stave off, to postpone aging can be fun—provided you try it with an open-minded attitude. Remember also that a negative attitude tells your age more than wrinkles do—the wrinkles one can count. Emotional well-being greatly, though not solely, depends upon an optimistic attitude, which is a cosmetic to the soul, while depression is the kind of cosmetic used by embalmers. And the type of depression that is a reaction to circumstances can be handled—as briefly discussed in the foregoing.

There are many examples of great men who have risen to prominence after they should have shut up shop according to the chronologic calendar. Paul von Hindenburg, the German general, was an obscure functionary at 66 until he was recalled at the outbreak of World War I and rose to greatness, successfully losing a war for the Germans. The great Louis Pasteur, who at 45 suffered a stroke and with it what he believed was the end of a useful life, suddenly embarked on a positive approach to his life, resumed his consuming interest in his work, and completed the most important research in the next 20 years of his life—the treatment for rabies.

These men did not believe what the prophets of doom had to say, and in their lifetimes the life expectancy for man was less than 50 years.

People are reputed to be increasingly egotistical as they grow older. A great loss is suffered thereby, because it clouds their perception. The following quotation, from a source long forgotten, expresses the idea fully:

> The more egotistical and self-centered a person grows, the more his insight is reduced. *Insight is the common sense of the soul.* It follows therefore, that when your gaze is concentrated on yourself, you are oblivious of things around you. When we become less alert to others we lose much of the ability of insight into others due to being encapsulated in ourselves. It is not due to self-abnegation or altruism that we should be alert and aware of people around us, but due to intelligent self-interest.

CHAPTER 3

Other Faces of Aging

Age is a deadly disease. But few people become personally aware of its inexorable march until their 50s—at the time when the rate of aging becomes more difficult to slow down. The situation is further complicated by the fact that aging is a many-sided process. Perhaps thousands of events go on in the body that all together spell deterioration before death. While methods to halt aging are not at hand, various investigators have tried to study the implacable process of aging from different angles. Each may possibly shed some light on the complex puzzle; there is no single answer. There are multiple answers and we hope that the right answers may be in the mixture.

It is interesting to observe that there are two utterly stressful experiences to which man is subject: birth and aging. "Birth is the most endangering experience to which most individuals are ever exposed," according to Dr. Abraham Towbin (*Journal of the American Medical Association*, Aug. 30, 1971). He refers to mechanical damage and reduced oxygen availability in the process of birth.

The stress in birth can be cataclysmic and can mark an individual for life. But the stresses of aging start slowly, are progressive, and accelerate with time. The longer you live the more rapid and ineluctable the deterioration.

Many ideas have been proposed by medical researchers—and some have been experimentally tried—in order to gain an understanding of aging and, hence, to reduce its rate (that is, to retard its destructive qualities). We shall not go into a recitation of fads or into dramatic doings such as Serge Voronoff's transplantation of a chimpanzee's testicles into a man back in the 1920s in an attempt to enable him to recapture the sexual potency of his youth. But we shall summarize some findings which appear to have some validity and which have been repeated by other investigators. They may add pieces to help fill in some part of the incredibly complex puzzle of aging.

Undernutrition.

One of the comparatively recent experiments in aging was started in 1927 by Dr. Clive M. McCay. He found that by underfeeding rats he could increase their life span enormously—could almost double it. He tried this experiment to test his thesis that age is related to the rate of maturation—that the longer it takes an animal to mature into adulthood the greater its lifespan. His notion was also confirmed in reverse, for when his underfed and long-lived rats were put on a plentiful diet, they grew rapidly—and died. Whether death was due to the fact that they had already reached an age almost twice that of the regularly fed group (that had only a normal lifespan) or that they died from sudden access to unlimited food is not clear.

Subsequently, other experiments confirmed McCay's findings. These findings may have wide importance and do raise questions that have social, political, and economic import: Is the undernutrition in pockets of poverty a blessing in disguise since it may lengthen the lifespan? What good is a longer lifespan when the individual lives in poverty and deprivation? Does a longer lifespan also mean that the long-living individual retains his mental acuity? Since undernutrition retards the multiplication and growth of newer cells, does the underfed individual ever develop a mental capacity comparable to that of the so-called average man?

These questions are easier to ask than to answer.

Another point bears mention, and that is the applicability to man of findings in rats and other animals. Results obtained in other animals cannot automatically be applied to man. Thoughtful study does, however, show that there are often parallels between man and other animals. For example, when a given condition—say, muscle abnormality—is produced in many species of animals when they are deprived of a given vitamin, it can clearly be tested in man. Most of our nutritional knowledge is obtained from tests in rats and other animals. But it must be further tested in man.

And outside of war, man is not expendable. Hence, it is not possible to subject man to the same deprivations or other stresses to which animals can be subjected in the search for answers.

How can the finding that undernutrition—learned by experience in animals—leads to longer life be practically applied to man? It is difficult for an individual to do so, but a few guidelines may help you: (1) reduce your caloric intake, especially of starches and sugars; (2) increase the protein part of your diet; (3) take a sufficient variety and amount of accessory food factors—the vitamins—as well as minerals. As we shall see later, it may be especially desirable—especially for the older person—to have an adequate intake of vitamin E. But a recommendation of reduced food intake across-the-board may be an oversimplification because aging people need supporting foods, especially amino acids found in proteins, though they can usually do with fewer calories.

Other theories of aging.

There are a number of theories on why aging occurs; some are briefly outlined here:

Waste products theory: The accumulation of certain waste products of metabolism interfere with certain ongoing reactions in the body. Metabolism is the sum total of the events that go on in the body in its normal functions of converting food to energy and of performing other functions to retain health.

Speed rate theory: The greater the rate of metabolism, the shorter the lifespan—"burning up" too quickly. This also means that the more you eat, the more fuel your body must "burn up," and the more adjustments it must make down the line, such as disposing of metabolic waste.

Free radical theory: Portions break off from chemical compounds in the body. These portions, called free radicals, are highly reactive and enter into other reactions that accelerate aging. Vitamin E is an antioxidant, and it inhibits or helps neutralize the untoward effect of free radicals by acting as a shield against the oxidation and other chemical changes caused by free radicals.

Mutation theory: Age is accelerated when mutations, or molecular changes, occur in cells—for example, radiation from X rays or other sources encourages mutation.

Stress theory: The more stress you put on the body,

the greater the breakdown; this is also related to the speed rate theory. Stresses include disease, extremes of temperature, and inadequate nutrition. Young animals adapt to stress better than do older ones.

Cross-linkage theory: Age is a process when the various molecules interconnect—or cross-link—with others in the tissues. The efficiency of the functioning of tissues that have a substantial amount of cross-linked molecules is reduced.

Protein synthesis theory: "Mistranslation" of nucleic acids DNA and RNA occurs when an enzyme, RNA polymerase, gives false instructions to an RNA messenger. The result—the mismatching of different RNA and DNA arrangements—produces anomalous patterns. These patterns are the blueprints for building proteins. Faulty blueprints produce faulty buildings.

Oxidation theory: All things age and become less efficient upon oxidation, which is the chemical process wherein oxygen enters a molecule and changes its structure and function. For example, a dried-up rubber tube has become oxidized, has lost its elasticity, has become brittle, and breaks under even a minor stress. The use of vitamin E is based largely on the oxidation theory.

Each of these theories may have some part in helping us to understand the complex phenomenon that aging represents.

Levels of aging.

According to the eminent research scientist, Dr. A. L. Tappel of the University of California at Davis, aging has a timetable. One degenerative change after another appears in sequence. And reviewing the evidence, it appears to be true.

Where do these changes start? At different levels. And they ascend until deterioration approaches completion. What is the timing? It follows the changes at each level.

The first level at which deterioration proceeds is at the molecular level. This is where molecular reactions take place—for example, this is where free radicals, which are highly reactive parts of molecules, wreak havoc by causing oxidation or peroxidation of the partially unsaturated fatty acids (lipids) in the tissues. Remember that *un*saturated fats are particularly liable to saturation or oxidation, and that attack by the free radicals further increases their oxidation. And free radicals can change proteins so that the proteins cannot perform their function in the body economy. The need for an antioxidant—something to hinder oxidation—is manifest.

The second level where oxidation damage continues is at the cell level. Various parts of cells perform a function—in synchronization with other transactions—such as the function of the mitochondria, the powerpacks, in energy metabolism. A cell cannot fully function when part of it has been degraded by oxidation.

The third level of damage is at the organ level. Organs are composed of large numbers of specialized cells organized to perform a function. When many cells in an organ are damaged, the function of the organ is impaired. The damaged organ then cannot perform its function, cannot dispose of its waste metabolites, and cannot renew itself. These changes are initiated and surely accentuated by peroxidation of lipids.

Antioxidants.

There are various *kinds* of biochemical changes

which are associated with aging. Oxidation is one of them. *But the process of oxidation is one that takes place at many levels of structure and function.* Fortunately it can be inhibited by an antioxidant—such as vitamin E. That vitamin acts as a fatty "free radical trap," just as vitamin C acts as an aqueous free radical trap. In fact, Dr. Tappel reminds us that vitamins E and C work synergistically, that ". . . the biochemistry of vitamin E deficiency and the aging process run parallel . . .," and that further investigation should continue to find even better ways of using other antioxidants as well as vitamin E.

Vitamin E is believed by many scientists to markedly aid in keeping healthy. This belief is not in conflict with theories of aging—that is, part of each of the eight theories mentioned above may well be true. In that context, vitamin E can still play an important role in maintaining health and hopefully in retarding aging or the loss of healthy functions in many parts of the body. And probably the role of vitamin E is also that of a catalyst.

Vitamin E is an antioxidant; that is, it protects other substances against oxidation and helps to avert or reduce changes produced by oxidation. Antioxidants have clearly increased the lifespan of rats. How vitamin E applies to humans is not as clear as it is in other animals, though if there is enough vitamin E in the human system certain good things happen; for example, the unsaturated fatty acids are protected from oxidation. And tissues contain unsaturated fatty acids among other lipids.

An unsaturated compound is one that still has space in the molecule to take on another element, such as oxygen or hydrogen. An unsaturated fatty acid can take on oxygen, and when it does, it is considered oxidized. (If it takes on hydrogen it is called hydrogenated—as hydrogenated fats, which are saturated fats.)

Thus, the unsaturated fatty acids are susceptible to oxidation. What prevents the acquisition of oxygen is an antioxidant—meaning a substance that works against oxidation.

There are other antioxidants—butylated hydroxytoluene, a food additive, is one example—and some are even more effective than vitamin E. However, the outstanding feature of vitamin E resides in these facts: (1) it is a natural antioxidant; that is, it is found in nature (though it can be synthetically produced) and is widely distributed in the animal and vegetable kingdoms; and (2) it is nontoxic; no poisoning with tocopherol was ever reported in man though given in large doses for long periods. There are other antioxidants especially used in animals which do obliterate some of the signs of vitamin E deprivation, but none removes all the signs that vitamin E does.

Of course, this does not mean that it is desirable to do away with oxygen in order to avoid oxidation. Oxygen is vital to life. Yet, the marvelous programming of the human body is such that, while it cannot live without oxygen, the body selectively reduces the amount of oxygen in places and functions where oxygen can do harm. Vitamin E helps the body to reduce the amount of oxygen when a function or metabolic transaction would be adversely affected. Thus vitamin E protects the fats (lipids) or other substances in the cells that would be damaged by oxygen.

Perhaps there is logic in this phenomenon. With aging there is oxidation—even in such inanimate substances as rubber. And therewith, the need for vitamin E is greater in older animals than in young ones. This has been demonstrated in rats. Whether, or in what degree, it applies to man quantitatively is yet to be determined satisfactorily.

Dangers of oxidation.

In many happenings it is not possible to say if there is a cause-effect relationship—which is cause, which is effect. Many observations are made on the basis of association. For example, one finds increased oxidation in aging, and also in aging there is a destruction of tissue or certain membranes. Is the one the cause or the result of the other? It is not known. But a sufficient number of associations are present to suggest strongly that there is a link between oxidation and aging. For example, while it is not known if oxidation of fats is the result of aging or if causally it hastens aging, it is clear that oxidation is present and increases during aging.

Oxidation always goes on—normally. The question is one of rate, that is, the speed of oxidation. Antioxidants are not used to obliterate oxidation but to retard its rate or speed.

An example where oxygen is clearly harmful exists in retrolental fibroplasia, which is a condition of the eye producing blindness. It has been found to occur in premature babies that have been exposed to a high oxygen atmosphere to enable them to survive permanently.

Another example of the untoward effect of oxygen is in the use of hyperbaric chambers. These are closed units, containing oxygen under high pressure, in which persons with respiratory and other problems are placed. The changes that occur as a result of exposure to hyperbaric oxygen parallel those found in aging.

A recent report by Drs. Senior, Wessler, and Avioli in the *Journal of the American Medical Association* (Sept. 6, 1971) emphasizes that oxygen, though life-sustaining, can be toxic to the lungs especially when given in the large amounts often necessary in emergencies to support life. The hazard is greatly dependent upon the amount and the length of time during which oxygen is administered. Numerous enzyme functions can be brought to a standstill by such high oxygen administration, which may favor the formation of the dangerous free radicals. Other instances when high oxygen administration may be dangerous include the use of incubators for premature infants and of intensive care units, although here the great amounts of oxygen are usually life-saving.

The report of Drs. Senior, Wessler, and Avioli deals with damage to the lungs and to the whole respiratory apparatus produced by high oxygen tension. This is especially striking in view of the fact that Thomas Beddoes (a British physician of the 18th century who first used oxygen in medicine) and Antoine Lavoisier (the great French chemist also of the 18th century) independently observed and wrote about lung damage from oxygen.

These events emphasize the fact that man can live safely and comfortably only in a very narrow margin of safety. This refers to heat and cold as well as to the amount of oxygen he breathes. A low oxygen level (hypoxia) as well as a high oxygen level (hyperoxia) can each produce extensive damage and in severe deprivation or excess can kill.

Pigments associated with aging.

Another point of association is noteworthy. It concerns the development of certain pigments, called ceroids or lipofuscins, which are usually found in aging persons as well as in animals. These pigments increase during aging. And their presence is also seen in vitamin E deprivation. Though these pigments of age may be innocent debris or fallout—it is not known what their presence signifies—they do accumulate in the heart and (what is more important) in brain cells, upon aging. Dr. Bernard A. Strehler, of the University of Southern California, a respected authority on aging, concurs that age pigments such as ceroid predictably increase with aging of the human heart tissue. Strehler has long held that aging is a programmed deterioration, not just a wearing out of parts of the body.

Is the occurrence of these pigments both in aging and in vitamin E deprivation merely an accident? It happens too frequently to be dismissed. And these pigments are also produced in membranes through oxidation.

Vitamin E suppresses the peroxidative and deteriorative reactions of fats or lipids that are associated with aging. (The terms "peroxidation" and "oxidation" are used here interchangeably—peroxidation is a higher form of oxidation. For the purposes of this discussion they can be considered to be the same.) Since this is so, one might think that deprivation of vitamin E should be quickly noticeable.

But that is not the case.

Vitamin E deficiency.

Obvious signs of deficiency in man develop slowly. In animals they appear more rapidly and dramatically. Although it takes time for signs of deficiency to be clear and recognizable in man, often a year or more, the damage done by deprivation nonetheless occurs. Considering the fact that vitamin E is absorbed through the lymph, is stored in the liver, and is found in most organs in man—including kidneys, lungs, pancreas, heart, spleen, liver, and muscles, with the highest levels in the adrenal glands, the testes, and the pituitary—it becomes apparent how widespread the damage can be through deprivation of vitamin E.

The first sign of a lack of vitamin E may be a certain type of blood destruction. Or an excess urinary excretion of creatine, a substance involved in muscle contraction, which suggests a metabolic dysfunction in the muscles. Or perhaps the deposition of ceroid age pigment. But the effects of deprivation that give no early signs may be more serious—we do not know.

There is the danger that by the time symptoms do appear, after a number of years, damage may have already been done—that is, aging may have already occurred.

Deficiency of vitamin E may develop from (1) an inadequate intake of vitamin E (such as eating food lacking in vitamin E), (2) malabsorption (see Chapter 4), which is reduced ability of the body to absorb fats and vitamin E from the intestine, (3) or an increased intake of polyunsaturated fatty acids.

How much vitamin E?

What is the daily requirement of vitamin E? Even though certain guidelines have been set forth by the Food and Nutrition Board of the National Research Council (see Chapter 10), the actual amount needed depends upon how much of the polyunsaturated fatty acids is taken in the daily diet. The more polyunsaturated fatty acids that are taken in food, the more vitamin E is needed, because a portion of the vitamin E is used in protecting the unsaturation of the unsaturated fatty acids. Also, food processing destroys a considerable amount of vitamin E. Polyunsaturated fatty acids are found in margarine and in corn and other vegetable oils. There are no polyunsaturated fatty acids in olive oil and coconut oil.

This does not mean that oils containing polyunsaturated fatty acids should be dropped from the diet—only that more vitamin E should be taken to make up for what is used up by the polyunsaturated fatty acids. Polyunsaturated fats are vital in the body economy.

Age is a gradual but general deterioration in virtually

all organs—including but not limited to the brain, heart and vessels of circulation, muscles, and kidneys. In animals, the deficiency of vitamin E shows a greater variety of pathological conditions, dysfunctions, diseases, or disorders than the deficiency of any other single vitamin. It affects the reproductive, muscular, skeletal, circulatory, and respiratory systems and produces disturbances of the liver, the kidneys, and the blood.

The parallel to man is logical and quite possible.

For that reason symptoms of vitamin E deprivation in older animals—and presumably in man—are harder to detect; these symptoms can easily be confused with the pathological changes associated with aging. The gravity of the situation becomes more apparent when it is realized that these changes—clearly in animals, and also presumably in man—*are not reversible* if they have existed undetected for varying lengths of time. Therefore it is not surprising that gerontologists Richard J. Passwater and Paul A. Welker of the American Gerontological Research Laboratories believe that the use of vitamin E, in addition to other antioxidants, can lengthen the lifespan in man by five to ten years. Their theory is an integrated one and includes the mistranslation of DNA and RNA mentioned earlier. In addition, they believe that increasing the vitamin B complex, vitamin C, with vitamin E, plus sulfur-containing aminoacids and several minerals can add 30 years of useful life. Dr. A. L. Tappel apparently is quite optimistic as to the importance of nutrient elements when he says that "there is no theoretical reason why our lives cannot be extended using protectors against the deterioration of fats." He found a 50% increase in the lifespan in mice that were fed large amounts of vitamin E.

Oxidation, or peroxidation, of fats has nothing to do with obesity! Even thin people normally have lipids—fat in tissue.

Free radicals.

How vitamin E works—namely, the mechanism of action of antioxidants—is not known. It is conjectured by Dr. William A. Pryor, professor of chemistry at Louisiana State University, in his thoughtful work on free radicals, that antioxidants hasten or increase the formation of the microsomal enzymes, which are the *power-packs* in the cell.

The oxidation theory is closely linked to the free radical theory. Free radicals are electrically charged parts of molecules from which certain atoms have sprung off—after which the radicals are highly active in the search to mate with another stable connection. If they make a connection with an unsaturated fatty acid, they oxidize, or peroxidize, the latter.

Free radicals may do other damage. Connecting with other radicals they may form new substances—*monster proteins*—not useful to the cell. In the body what is not useful is detrimental.

In deficiency of an antioxidant or of vitamin E, radiation will produce free radicals, which would then rearrange and have free rein to do damage. Radiation is one way in which free radicals are formed.

Thus, the following conditions resemble one another: (1) damage from radiation—with its discharge of free radicals; (2) deterioration associated with age; and (3) deficiency of vitamin E.

Is it a wonder that vitamin E has been considered the age vitamin? If vitamin E is related to aging, then an inadequate intake or supply of vitamin E may well take productive years from life. And vitamin E is not synthesized by the body—it must be taken either through food or by ingestion of vitamin E preparations. Although actual vitamin E deficiency in man is infrequent, it appears that more than a mere subsistence amount is necessary to perform its many tasks, particularly to act as an antioxidant shield against free radicals.

Polyunsaturated fatty acids.

Another substance lurks on the stage on which the action of vitamin E takes place—that substance is polyunsaturated fatty acids, and it is both friend and enemy: friend, because vitamin E, being fat soluble, is absorbed from fat; and enemy, in that polyunsaturated fatty acids in corn oil and other polyunsaturated oils take away some of the antioxidant property from vitamin E. Vitamin E also comes to the aid of polyunsaturated fatty acids—to prevent their degradation (that is, their change into a noxious form by the action of radiation or free radicals upon them). Vitamin E prevents such damage to polyunsaturated fatty acids by protecting them from peroxidation.

The subject of aging and well-being is increasingly being considered from the viewpoint of antioxidants, as well as from that of cross-linkage and DNA-RNA mistranslation—among the aging theories discussed earlier. The coming years will doubtlessly see an even greater concern with adequate function while aging.

The desire for longevity and man's preoccupation with age were acutely recognized even by the ancient Romans. Terence, a Roman poet who flourished before 150 B.C., bemoaned that old age is a disease by itself (*Senectus ipsa morbus est*). And Cicero, the great Roman statesman and orator of the first century B.C., expressed his insight into his contemporaries when he noted that no one is so old as to think that he does not have one more year of life (*Nemo enim est tam senex qui se annum non putet passe vivere*).

Conference on aging.

The Duttweiler Institute Conference on Aging, which met in Zurich, Switzerland, in the fall of 1971, was mainly concerned with the increase of the lifespan. (But a long life without well-being and retention of our faculties is pointless—it becomes a burden rather than a gift. Note the population of half-alive people in nursing homes, people whose lives are burdensome to all concerned, including themselves.) The conference assembled eminent researchers in aging who expressed their views, forecast research direction, and revealed results.

Outstanding interest was expressed by the participants in antioxidants and particularly in vitamin E. Other ideas on aging which were aired included the reduction of body temperature by drugs to hold off aging by Dr. Bernard A. Strehler (reminiscent of the speed rate theory, which holds that the greater the rate of metabolism the more quickly the organism ages or "burns out"); reduction of caloric intake by Dr. Alex Comfort, internationally known British gerontologist (reminiscent of McCay's mice mentioned earlier); the cross-linkage theory; and replacement of aging nerve and muscle cells (requiring a spare parts organ bank, which probably will not come for a hundred years).

But apparently the greatest thrust was concern with antioxidants: butylated hydroxytoluene, a chemical used as a food additive to prevent spoilage of foods by oxidation, and vitamin E.

While no new ideas on just how vitamin E works were put forth at that conference, reaffirmations of current views of the functions of vitamin E were voiced. Hence, there was general agreement that vitamin E inhibits peroxidation of lipids. Accord was also expressed for the increased need for vitamin E now that more polyunsaturated oils are used in foods. The use of polyunsaturated oils dispenses with or reduces the intake of animal fats with their high cholesterol potential. But if polyunsaturated fatty acids from the oils are oxidized, free radicals or dienes can form, which are toxic, and vitamin E prevents the formation of such free radicals. It was also brought out that another reason for increasing the amount of vitamin E is that polyunsaturated oils use up vitamin E in the attempt to protect themselves from oxidation.

One important point resulting from that conference should be borne in mind: that the optimum time to begin using vitamin E is at the time when it will do most good—before aging takes a foothold. This would suggest that the ideal time to begin is the 20s or 30s. But the need for vitamin E actually begins with infancy.

Ozone.

We spoke of vitamin E as an antioxidant to protect against oxidation by oxygen. What about the *superoxygen,* namely, ozone?

Ozone is a form of oxygen with a tremendous wallop. Some notion can be gained by comparing the atomic notation for oxygen, which is O_2, with that of ozone. Ozone is O_3. Though similar to oxygen, it is a substance with more powerful effects than oxygen in degree and also in *kind*, as it has effects that oxygen does not.

For example, the lung damage done by smog is largely due to ozone, though sulfur dioxide contributes to the damage.

Drs. Tappel and Goldstein clearly report that the ". . . survival of rats exposed to 3 to 15 parts per million of ozone is decreased if the animal's supply of vitamin E is inadequate." What threatens survival is oxidation, or more properly, peroxidation of the tissues.

This same peroxidation occurs on exposure to X rays or to high levels of oxygen. Vitamin E protects mice against the effects of hyperbaric oxygen, that is, oxygen at high pressures.

Two sentinels stand guard against the metabolic cataclysms of oxidation and damage by free radicals. One is vitamin E—a fat-soluble antioxidant. The other is vitamin C—a water-soluble antioxidant.

Premature senility.

There is a dreadful condition in connection with aging that vitamin E probably cannot arrest—though in fact, as far as is now known, it has not been tried. The condition is progeria, a premature senility that can afflict the very young and literally make a boy of eight look like 80.

This condition of rapid aging occurs even before the child reaches puberty. In it, a child is buffeted by the physical and mental ravages of age; while he develops senile features, he does not develop the intellectual characteristics, such as wisdom, which at times come with age. In fact, the unfortunate child remains infantile, with milk teeth and without body hair. But the formations of the face and posture change into those of a grotesque old man.

This condition, a tremendously accelerated rate of aging, is caused by errors of metabolism. This is a state when one or more enzymes that are present in a body with normal metabolism fail to develop. The failure is genetically caused. Somewhere, in the fantastically complicated development of a fetus, nature slipped a cog.

Visionaries.

Vitamin E may turn out to be a vitamin with far-reaching social importance—depending on what future research will disclose. Being at one time touted as a cure-all may have caused resistance to looking at it seriously before the 1960s. The intrepid and farseeing investigators, such as K. S. Bishop, R. H. Bunnell, H. A. Evans, P. L. Harris, D. C. Herting, M. K. Horwitt, D. B. Menzel, H. M. Nitkowsky, R. J. Passwater, O. A. Roels, E. V. Shute, A. L. Tappel, P. A. Welker, and many others who painstakingly labored in the vineyard during the dark days of vitamin E, may have turned the tide.

Many creative people intuitively see the light at the end of the tunnel before any logical evidence has been worked out.

This concept brings to mind the words of the great mathematician Karl Friedrich Gauss (1777–1855) who said:

> I have had my solutions for a long time but I do not yet know how I am to arrive at them.

CHAPTER 4

Malabsorption

What is malabsorption? It is a failure of the system to absorb nutrition from the small intestine, where all absorption of food takes place. Malabsorption is impairment of the absorption of foods, minerals, and water. More specifically, the absorption of fats and fat-soluble vitamins—such as A, D, K, and of course vitamin E, also a fat-soluble vitamin—is impeded.

Malabsorption is related to or may include such conditions as nontropical sprue or celiac disease of children and cystic fibrosis of the pancreas. "Celiac" just means belly—it is an adjective for belly, and "celiac disease" merely means belly disease. But as commonly used it means a particular form of belly disease, a condition characterized by absorptive dysfunctions and especially by a passing of fatty stools. Fatty stools are recognized by their color and looseness and are due to the fact that fats are excreted rather than being partially absorbed. Cystic fibrosis of the pancreas is an inflammatory condition of the pancreas. This group of conditions is generally called the malabsorption syndrome.

Hence malabsorption is characterized by such conditions as fatty stools, a poorly nourished state leading to underweight, anemia, and excess excretion of creatine in the urine. Creatine is an amino acid normally found in the muscles. When a relatively large amount is excreted in the urine it may mean muscle disease or other troubles. That is the reason it is looked for in the attempt to find a diagnosis of a suspicious or puzzling condition.

Deficiency of vitamin E in healthy people in the United States has not been reported—perhaps that is one reason for their *relatively* healthy status. But that does not apply to people with symptoms of the malabsorption syndrome. In malabsorption there is a clear failure to absorb fats and principally those accessory nutrients found in fats—vitamins. That means vitamins A, D, E, and K. And if vitamin E, a fat-soluble vitamin, is not absorbed, it may lead to an added complication.

Children with cystic fibrosis fail to thrive. That would be expected if they do not absorb and utilize food. But many such children do reach adulthood—some even marry and have children, because women who have the malabsorption syndrome can reproduce. But amazingly, *the men are sterile*—there is no sperm in their ejaculate!

Reproduction.

Is there a relationship between men who have a malabsorption syndrome and cannot reproduce and the rats deprived of vitamin E who fail to reproduce? When female rats are deprived of vitamin E they can conceive, but the developing fetus is resorbed (which means, before it is fully grown it degenerates, and the resulting material is absorbed).

In fact, the first observation of the effect of vitamin

E was that it is indispensable to the fertility of rats. It was called a fertility vitamin in that context and for that reason. Most recently Drs. C. Raychaudhuri and I. D. Desai, of the Division of Human Nutrition of the University of British Columbia, reported that the sterility of female rats that have been deprived of vitamin E may well be due to the tissue damage in reproductive organs caused by peroxidation of fats. They observed that such animals had fat deposits in their bellies and deposits of ceroid pigment in the uterus and fallopian tubes—deposits that animals which were not deprived of vitamin E did not show. When vitamin E was given to the deprived rats for 60 days they resumed growth but remained sterile.

This analogy becomes more interesting when we consider that malabsorption in man may exhibit signs similar to those in animals when they are deprived of vitamin E: muscle weakness, deposition of ceroid (an age pigment), breakdown of red blood cells, and great excretion of creatine in the urine, which may be a sign of muscular dystrophy in animals.

Other investigators, including Drs. Nitkowsky, Tildon, Levin, and Gordon, from the departments of Pediatrics of the Sinai Hospital of Baltimore and the Johns Hopkins School of Medicine in Baltimore, studying tocopherol deficiency in infants and children, found that the biochemical changes in patients with cystic fibrosis of the pancreas resemble the changes in animals with vitamin E deficiency that have developed muscular dystrophy. They consider this finding to be a parallel and believe that the *counterpart* of animal deprivation of vitamin E can develop in man.

Impaired absorption.

This does not mean that vitamin E is the royal remedy for all symptoms of the malabsorption syndrome. Celiac syndrome in children can improve strikingly when wheat and other grains containing gluten are eliminated from the diet. Other measures are also necessary. But the role of vitamin E in the metabolism and absorption of fats in man is particularly clear, especially in view of the fact that various stresses increase the need for vitamins over that taken just for the prevention of a deficiency or over the amounts obtainable in food.

Steatorrhea—fatty stools—is a uniform finding in malabsorption. Dr. H. J. Binder and his associates at Yale University School of Medicine found that in a set of 55 patients with gastrointestinal disease, a full 30% had vitamin E deficiency. It is his belief that the presence of steatorrhea *due to any cause* was the one common factor in this group which were vitamin E deficient.

In fact, in malabsorption, when there is a low level of one substance, the absorption of related substances is often impeded. Thus, in children with cystic fibrosis, Dr. Mildred J. Bennett, of the Children's Hospital Medical Center of Northern California at Oakland, found that when vitamins A and E are given together, the levels of both vitamins A and E rise without increasing the daily dose of either vitamin, and that therewith the excessive creatine excretion in the urine is reduced.

Few diseases are of isolated importance—they often have ramifications in other systems of the body. Another example of this phenomenon is the case of animals in which vitamin E deficiency was induced—the deposition of ceroid was also found. And ceroid deposition in cells of the intestine has long been found in association with steatorrhea.

Is there a relationship between two events when they repeatedly occur together? Some signs suggest that there is. In the chapters on aging the phenomenon of association is discussed—when two symptoms repeatedly happen to be present at the same time they may be related. It does not always follow that one causes the other. But if a cause and effect relationship cannot be demonstrated in the association of two events occurring together, its study may be a highly fertile undertaking. After association is observed, the next step in a scientific investigation is correlation—that is, to find out if such two associated events dovetail and give further evidence of a cause and effect relationship.

That there is such a correlation was shown by Drs. Loesel, Schnitzer, and Herting from the Department of Pathology of the University of Michigan. They report that vitamin E deficiency, as shown by low tocopherol levels in the blood, can occur in patients with longstanding malabsorption syndrome. These two events—malabsorption and vitamin E deficiency—do not occur until the signs of malabsorption have been present for about two years. But the fact that they do occur is important, as it demonstrates one probable cause and effect relationship.

This slow process of degradation is not a blessing. Dr. M. K. Horwitt, St. Louis University School of Medicine, who is among the outstanding investigators of vitamin E, points out that once degradation (peroxidation) due to vitamin E deprivation has occurred, it will probably take an abnormally large amount of vitamin E to inhibit further peroxidation. Note, nothing is said about reversing the process—but only about preventing further damage.

This book is about vitamin E, not malabsorption. The purpose of this chapter is merely to point out the intrinsic role of vitamin E in dysfunctions of intestinal absorption and of metabolism of food, which is part of the malabsorption syndrome.

A substance that is touted to be good for everything often turns out to be good for nothing. That platitude has merit—as is often the case with platitudes. But one must look beyond platitudes and clichés. Some people depend on clichés because they have no other information.

The search for truth goes on not only in science, but in every aspect of human endeavor. If we stop, we will be overwhelmed by ignorance. Alfred North Whitehead, the great English philosopher and mathematician, gave us an insight in our search for truths:

> There are no whole truths; all truths are half-truths. It is trying to treat them as whole truths that plays the devil.*

* *Dialogues of Alfred North Whitehead,* 1954.

CHAPTER 5

Polyunsaturated Fatty Acids and the Liver

Since about 1960 there has been a nationwide push to overcome or reduce atherosclerosis. This is a condition in which there is an accumulation of a soft fatty mass, predominantly cholesterol, in the walls of the arteries. Atherosclerosis is dangerous because the deposition of cholesterol and other fatty materials in the arteries reduces their diameter or width. The reduced diameter impedes the unrestricted circulation of the blood. The parallel can be made to a water pipe that is rust encrusted—the rust impedes the flow of water.

The deposition of cholesterol is associated with heart attack. To reduce the frequency of heart attacks—believed to be due to cholesterol accumulation in the arteries—it was believed that the dietary intake of cholesterol should be reduced. That concept was attractive and logical and hence became a persuasive one.

Reducing cholesterol intake.

As a result, many studies were begun, notably the

famous Framingham, Massachusetts, study in which the diet was substantially reduced in cholesterol content. That was indeed a logical step: but not all that is logical is necessarily true. The reason that the cholesterol hypothesis may not be the answer to atherosclerosis, is because the deposition of cholesterol in the body is triggered by several other metabolic events. In other words, the body makes its own cholesterol even if a virtually cholesterol-free diet is eaten. And bear in mind that cholesterol is necessary in the body. It is the keystone to the formation of certain hormones—the sex hormones and the adrenocortical steroid hormones. Cholesterol, like hormones, is necessary but it depends on the place—in the lining of the arteries it's no good.

But to reduce the intake of cholesterol, people reduced in their diet foods which are rich in cholesterol. More particularly, the intake of dairy foods—milk and butter—as well as eggs and animal fats was considerably curtailed. To that end, people used skim milk instead of whole milk, margarine instead of butter, and polyunsaturated vegetable oils, such as corn or safflower oil, instead of animal fats or vegetable shortening. Margarine also is made with unsaturated vegetable oils. In fact, the intake of polyunsaturated vegetable oils—with their polyunsaturated fatty acids (linoleic acid among others)—became virtually an obsession. (Shortening fats are also made from vegetable oils, but in the process of being hardened they become saturated, not unsaturated fats.)

But it was forgotten that the greater the intake of polyunsaturated oils with their polyunsaturated fatty acids, the greater the need for vitamin E!

In fact, as long ago as 1927, Drs. H. A. Evans and G. O. Burr found that the wheat germ oil containing only small amounts of vitamin E that they successfully fed to their rats to prevent sterility, became ineffective for that purpose when the amount of lard in the carefully measured rations was increased. Lard contains an appreciable amount of polyunsaturated fatty acids. And the more polyunsaturated acids that were ingested, the more vitamin E was needed. Polyunsaturates had upset the balance.

This means that a vitamin E deficiency can be produced or made worse by feeding enough polyunsaturated fatty acids; the greater the intake of polyunsaturated fatty acids, the greater the need for vitamin E.

However, since polyunsaturated vegetable oils actually do contain vitamin E, how can a vitamin E deficiency be produced? That was a puzzling question until it was resolved by the finding that the polyunsaturated oils utilize and consume their vitamin E to protect their unsaturation—the vitamin E is then not available for its antioxidant effect for the tissues. More particularly, there is too little vitamin E present in polyunsaturated fats to perform both tasks, namely to protect their unsaturation and to act as an antioxidant to prevent peroxidation of fats in the tissues.

One of the pioneers in vitamin E study, Dr. Philip L. Harris, found that at least 0.6 milligram of alpha-tocopherol is necessary to protect each gram of polyunsaturated fatty acids taken in the form of vegetable oils, for otherwise vitamin E becomes depleted in the body. Since it is calculated that the average daily consumption of polyunsaturated fatty acids is 24 grams, 14 milligrams of vitamin E are needed daily. This is the origin of the expression "vitamin E/PUFA (polyunsaturated fatty acids) ratio 0.6:1." And the more polyunsaturated fatty acids you take in food, the greater the need for vitamin E.

If polyunsaturated oils remain a staple in the American diet, it appears sound to assure an extra intake of vitamin E to avoid its depletion in the body. That point was made as long ago as 1961 by Drs. Kingsbury and Ward, two British doctors. The same conclusion was reaffirmed 10 years later by Dr. Nicholas R. DiLuzio, professor of physiology at Tulane University School of Medicine. (Dr. DiLuzio has actually amplified these findings, as we shall discuss later.) Therefore, because of the need that polyunsaturated fatty acids have for vitamin E, they avidly grasp it to prevent their own oxidation. But that can leave enzymes and nucleic acids without protection against attack by free radicals (see Chapter 3), leading to their degradation. Vitamin E provides that protection since it acts as a shield against oxidation.

Dienes in the liver.

Carbon tetrachloride is well known both as a dry cleaner and as a serious poison to the liver. It is striking to note that vitamin E protects against liver damage by carbon tetrachloride! This was found accidentally by Dr. DiLuzio: when studying liver damage in alcoholics, he came upon a group of substances in fat metabolism called dienes. A diene, which is a hydrocarbon (containing hydrogen and carbon), is an unsaturated compound. As such, it has double bonds, that is, places in the molecule where a new atom can be acquired. Such compounds are quite active or reactive. A diene has two unsaturated bonds or two places where saturation can take place. These dienes were in the lipids (fat)—where they can easily oxidize or peroxidize those lipids. This does not mean that the dienes are free radicals—but in some ways they act like free radicals mentioned earlier.

The significance of this finding is that the dienes are more easily changed into peroxidized fats in the absence of vitamin E. When the people under study were given vitamin E, their level of dienes in the blood was lowered. And the antioxidant effect was increased. When those people stopped taking vitamin E, their antioxidant level was decreased and the diene level increased—a clear indication of the effect of vitamin E in reducing the peroxidation of fats.

Polyunsaturated fats are useful in the diet. But the adage that "if a little bit is good, a lot is much better" simply is not true. Few things are black or white.

The question of unsaturated fats is closely related to the role of vitamin E in nutrition generally. It is in nutrition too, that there was resistance to the recognition of vitamin E for decades. That is all the more deplorable because deficiency in vitamin E is most harmful to the young growing animal—it is in youth that the protective effects of vitamin E can be most useful.

We recall the concept but not the origin of the following quotation which applies to this topic:

> We are always courageous enough
> to sacrifice the young.

CHAPTER 6

Respiration and Pollution

Environmental pollution is a fact. It is a problem in most parts of the world. The hazards are the same, only the pollutants may differ.

Air pollution is commonly defined as the presence of gaseous or particulate matter, arising from man's activities, which is discharged into the air in such a large volume or at such a rapid rate that it cannot be diffused quickly enough and therefore hangs in the air as a fog or smog. There are also naturally occurring pollutants that can harm man, such as ozone or cosmic rays. The latter also convert part of the exhaust from airplanes into ozone. With natural pollutants, too, it is a matter of quantity and rate of production in the air and the speed of dissipation.

Various pollutants can affect man—nitrogen oxides, sulfur dioxide, and ozone are examples of gaseous pollutants. They are partially responsible for the lung damage done by smog. They impair man's ability to breathe and oxygenate—but that is not the total damage they can do, for they can also create changes in the tissues of the respiratory tract by peroxidation. One of the manifestations of such changes may be emphysema (which, however, can also be due to other causes).

It would be idle to hope that we can scrub our air to make it pure. It is not realistic in the light of increasing industrialization. At best, pollution can be only reduced. However, the damage done by lifelong exposure to low concentrations of pollutants will still be noxious.

Role of vitamin E.

Vitamin E may play a key role here for two reasons: (1) by acting as a protective antioxidant in the tissues and (2) by protecting vitamin A, which is necessary for the health of the delicate respiratory membranes and other tissues. These were the findings disclosed by Drs. Roehm, De Lucca, Menzel, and Hadley in the Symposium on Pollution and Lung Biochemistry sponsored by Batelle-Northwest Institute in June 1970, as reported in *Chemical & Engineering News* under the title "Vitamins A and E Help Maintain Lung Health."

Vitamin E interposes an antioxidant shield against the destructive oxidizing effects of ozone and nitrogen dioxide. Again, the mechanism by which this takes place is by quenching or reducing the effect of free radicals (see Chapter 3), which oxidize polyunsaturated fatty acids in the tissues to form an aldehyde, malonylaldehyde, which poisons certain enzyme systems. In fact, malonylaldehyde is a danger, according to the cross-linkage theory of aging, if it degrades DNA, one of the nucleic acids of which every living thing is composed.

Experiments in which rats were exposed to deadly concentrations of ozone and nitrogen dioxide showed clearly that those protected with vitamins A and E lived about twice as long as the unprotected ones, according to the redoubtable Dr. A. L. Tappel. The rats under experiment were in a cage in which they breathed air containing specific amounts of these noxious gases for specified periods.

Does this mean that everyone should load up with vitamin E or they will die of breathing polluted air? Not necessarily at all. The final results are not in—research work is continuously being done. But in the light of results obtained thus far, it does indeed appear to be prudent to be sure of an adequate intake of vitamin E. Everyone must weigh the cost he wishes to expend for vitamin E against the probable good that research thus far has disclosed. Even if the results of research are still tentative, it appears that enough positive good has been discovered to merit vitamin E's serious consideration for health.

The following quotation, applicable here, has been variously ascribed both to William Collins (1721–1759), English poet, and Prince Otto von Bismarck (1815-1898), German statesman:

> A prudent person profits from his own experience, but a wise man profits from the experience of others.

CHAPTER 7

Circulation in the Legs

As a man ages, the circulation in his legs is often blocked. This is due to thickening as well as to loss of elasticity of the arteries. This condition is called peripheral vascular disease, as it refers to impeded circulation in the blood vessels in the periphery of the body (the legs). A variety of this condition is called intermittent claudication. Claudication means limping—hence intermittent claudication means merely that a person with that condition has episodes of limping or lameness. Upon walking pain and lameness occur, whereupon the person so affected has to stop and rest. After a few minutes rest, walking can be resumed—then the lameness recurs.

Improvement in this condition is measured by the increased distance an individual can walk before he is obliged to stop. In peripheral vascular conditions many investigators—especially the redoubtable pioneer in vitamin E therapy, Dr. Evan V. Shute, who introduced the treatment—report most encouraging results. The basis for the use of vitamin E in peripheral vascular disease rests on its antithrombotic effect—its antagonism to blood clots.

Recent studies include those of Dr. W. M. Toone, of the Department of Surgery of the Veterans Hospital of Victoria, British Columbia, who reports favorably on the use of vitamin E in arteriosclerotic peripheral vascular disease. But he also used other methods of treatment, and therefore the effect cannot be solely or definitely attributed to vitamin E.

A very recent report by Drs. H. T. G. Williams, D. Fenna, and R. A. Macbeth, of the Department of Surgery of the University of Alberta Hospital of Edmonton, Alberta, who carefully designed a research study with safeguarded controls, such as the use of placebos, does confirm that a group of patients with intermittent claudication were helped appreciably with doses of 400 milligrams of vitamin E given four times a day for several months. Other forms of peripheral vascular disease were not improved.

The eminent Dr. Alton Ochsner of the Ochsner Clinic of New Orleans, who like any surgeon, is concerned about the development of blood clots after an operation, believes that in addition to other measures vitamin E prevents thrombosis, or clotting. He wisely emphasizes that thrombosis and thromboembolism (a clot that travels) are better prevented than treated. Thrombophlebitis, which is clotting in the veins of the leg, is one danger in peripheral vascular disease. Vitamin E is used on the basis of reducing the clottability of the blood—not as a vasodilator, which dilates blood vessels.

When we learn better how vitamin E works—or even fails to work—in this group of diseases our understanding of the effect of vitamin E in other conditions will be enlarged as well. An editorial in the June 15, 1963, issue of the conservative and famous British medical journal, *The Lancet*, expresses the opinion that despite the mixed career of vitamin E, alpha-tocopherol, its most potent constituent, ". . . may yet gain a place in the conservative treatment of the mildly ischemic limb." Ischemia is a reduced circulation. If a substance is thought to have hope in the "conservative" treatment of a condition, it may well have arrived to take a serious place in therapy.

Oliver Wendell Holmes (1809-1894) famous American author, often reflected on and philosophized on the core of knowledge:

> The best part of our knowledge is that which teaches us where knowledge leaves off and ignorance begins. Nothing more clearly separates a vulgar from a superior mind, than the confusion in the first between the little that it truly knows on the one hand, and what it half knows and what it thinks it knows, on the other.

CHAPTER 8

Vitamin E and Muscle

There is an immense accumulation of evidence that animals deprived of vitamin E develop disease of the skeletal muscles. This is the type of muscle (also called voluntary, or striped, or striated muscle), connected at each end to bone, that enables movement to take place and through which "muscle power" is exerted. The damage to those muscles in vitamin E deficiency is extensive. In fact, vitamin E deprivation in rabbits produces a muscular dystrophy from which rabbits die in three weeks.

No such dramatic analogue exists in man, though vitamin E deprivation also affects him.

But one point in this problem has immense research value: skeletal muscles are voluntary muscles, subject to movement at will, while all other muscles are involuntary, not subject to movement at will. The one exception is the heart, which is made of the same fibers as are the skeletal muscles, though the heart is not subject to movement at will.*

Further work may possibly explain the reported role of vitamin E on the human heart, which is made of the same type of muscle fibers that in animals respond so dramatically to vitamin E. It is a pity indeed that no extensive, well-controlled studies on the effect of vitamin E in muscle have been reported. Such studies may explain much. The beaten path does not produce determinative results. Eric A. Johnston, at one time chairman of the U.S. Chamber of Commerce, put it epigrammatically:

> Beaten paths are for beaten men.

* But even that may not be so, when we consider the role of transcendental meditation in slowing the heart, or in influencing at will other functions which have heretofore been believed not to be controlled at will. The trouble is that we have to reckon with things which we do not know exist.

CHAPTER 9

Vitamin E and Blood

So dependable is the relationship of vitamin E to blood that a test for vitamin E deficiency is done by observing its effect on blood. It is called the erythrocyte hemolysis test. The test is based on the disruption of the red blood cell—called the erythrocyte—when brought into contact with an oxidizing agent. The oxidizing agent used in this test is hydrogen peroxide. In the event of a deficiency or a low level of vitamin E in the blood, the red blood cell ruptures and falls apart, or is hemolyzed. This test has been a road marker orienting researchers in vitamin E.

Other tests are also available; they differ in their responsiveness and in what aspect of vitamin E activity they measure. While the erythrocyte hemolysis test is used in animals in vitamin E research, it is particularly suitable for use in man—as a *live* test to show if the patient is vitamin E deficient. It is used in adults, but is particularly suitable for premature infants (preemies) and full-term babies.

Infants.

By the use of the erythrocyte hemolysis test, it was found that the vitamin E level in blood is often low in babies and, more particularly, that premature infants are likely to suffer from vitamin E deficiency. One reason for the frequent low level of vitamin E in preemies is that vitamin E does not pass the placental barrier between the mother and the child she is carrying.

If vitamin E deficiency is found, it can be overcome by administration of the vitamin. Premature infants respond strikingly. A dietary change may also be necessary to assure the continuous presence of vitamin E in the diet. For example, skim (low-fat) milk, which is often used in infants' diets, contains virtually no vitamin E. The supplementation of the diet with extra vitamin E is particularly necessary in such infants since the presence of polyunsaturated fatty acids in infant foods from vegetable oils further increases the need for vitamin E. Drs. Ritchie, Fish, McMasters, and Grossman, of the University of California–San Francisco Medical Center, affirming that a *common* cause of anemia and edema in infants is vitamin E deficiency, offer the reminder that the necessary presence of iron in an infant's formula destroys what trace of vitamin E is in the formula. Their investigations showed that the total amount of body stores of vitamin E in a full-term infant is only 20 milligrams and that in a premature infant it is an incredibly low 3 milligrams! Similar findings in infants weighing approximately 3.5 pounds, but not in those less than 3.5 pounds, were reported by Drs. Gross and Guilford of the Case Western Reserve University School of Medicine. Premature infants weighing 3.5 pounds or more responded to administration of vitamin E, but those weighing less than 3.5 pounds did not.

Older children.

Other types of anemia in older children have been reported by Dr. J. S. Dinning of the University of Arkansas School of Medicine to respond to vitamin E—which he considers in these instances a blood-building (hematopoietic) agent. In his investigation in Jordan, children low in vitamin E, who had large, immature blood cells (megaloblastic anemia) and symptoms of kwashiorkor (a nutritional disease of severely undernourished children, particularly found in Africa), responded to an adequate intake of vitamin E. Other investigations on vitamin E deficiency and its relation to hemolysis—among which is the scholarly study by Dr. Richard B. Goldbloom of the Montreal Children's Hospital and the Department of Pediatrics of McGill University—virtually reiterate the several findings reported above.

The erythrocyte hemolysis test merely shows that the red blood cells of vitamin E deficient animals and of man—but not the red blood cells of those not deficient—are hemolyzed, or fall apart, when brought into contact with hydrogen peroxide. By this test, levels of vitamin E in the blood below 0.5 milligrams for every 100 cc's are considered abnormal. This should not be construed to mean that vitamin E deficient adults will suddenly get hemolysis. This is not the case. But they may possibly develop other troubles.

In fact, while it is not fully known what the erythrocyte hemolysis test shows, it is clear that in vitamin E deficiency the antioxidant effect is low—the vitamin does not protect against the ravages of peroxidation. That is clearly demonstrated by the test, which creates hemolysis when such vitamin E deficient blood is brought in contact with an oxidizing agent—hydrogen peroxide. That little stress is enough to break up a red cell that does not have the antioxidant protection of vitamin E.

Many other questions are raised in this connection: (1) What is the relation between vitamin E level in the plasma (blood) and that in the tissues? (2) What other property of vitamin E, in addition to the antioxidant effect, is being measured? (3) In what other conditions, responsive to vitamin E, can the test be applied with confidence? (4) How does the test respond in the presence of sickle-cell anemia, which is a disease of the blood exclusively in Negroes, when there is no vitamin E deficiency?

There are many other questions which researchers in vitamin E probably are considering. Research takes a long time because one must reflect as to the possible significance a finding may have even before research is undertaken.

Possible uses of biological antioxidants such as vitamin E for other forms of diseases of the blood may be found in the near future. One such use is in a group of serious diseases called errors of metabolism, or hereditary metabolic diseases.

Errors of metabolism.

Errors of metabolism arise when there is a genetic lack of a certain enzyme or a block in the conversion of a given enzyme. For example, it is well known that people differ from each other. Some are even more *unequal* than others. In these *different* people, it seems that the genetic makeup slipped a cog in that, among other differences, they lack a "normal" enzyme to act as a link in the metabolic chain. For instance, the well-known condition, phenylketonuria, or PKU, is one in which infants fail to thrive and become mentally retarded owing to a lack of an enzyme. Since that enzyme is not present, it cannot convert the normally present amino acid, phenylalanine, into tyrosine. Hence, phenylalanine accumulates and turns into an aberrant substance known as phenylpyruvic acid. The missing enzyme, which is named phenylalanine hydroxylase, normally converts phenylalanine into tyrosine.

This is nature's error—it constitutes an error of metabolism of the amino acids. Errors of metabolism of substances other than amino acids also exist, some of which manifest themselves in genetically transmitted blood diseases.

Another such error of nature is a deficiency of an enzyme in the red blood cells called glucose 6-phosphate dehydrogenase, usually shortened to G6PD. When an individual has this condition, he may be usually well until he takes certain drugs to which he is explosively intolerant. It is not the drug per se that creates the problem; it only occurs when certain drugs meet a susceptible individual. Among such drugs are those against malaria, the sulfonamides, as well as certain other drugs. These drugs can trigger a blood-destroying (hemolytic) anemia, which means that the red blood cells are destroyed. The reason this happens is that when the red blood cells of a sensitive individual are challenged by such drugs, they speed up their oxygen consumption—they use up their oxygen at a highly rapid rate and fall apart.

Porphyria, which was mentioned earlier, is also a so-called error of metabolism. In that condition, certain pigments called porphyrins are overproduced because of a defect in certain enzymes in the body. The symptoms of the various kinds of porphyria are associated with an excretion of porphyrins in the urine.

While vitamin E has never been used in these conditions, as far as we know, it is possible that future research may find that the rapid oxygen consumption may be considerably reduced by a safe antioxidant, such as vitamin E.

Another form of blood destruction—though not as severe as hemolytic anemia—was noted in the blood of astronauts obliged to live in the oxygen-rich atmosphere of the Gemini spacecraft. In subsequent space explorations the administration of vitamin E prevented the parallel development of anemia.

At this stage a breadth of imagination must be the first prerequisite to further work in the niche of vitamin E investigation. Such a state of affairs is probably what Albert Einstein (1879–1955) had in mind when he flatly said:

> Imagination is more important than knowledge.

CHAPTER 10

Vitamin E in Nutrition

We are alert to the effect of drugs. We react to the term "habit-forming" as if it were a pestilence in all its contexts, when actually we have been conditioned against the bad *effects* of habit formation only as to drugs. Reacting thoughtlessly to the idea of habit formation, we may overlook the fact that many good practices—such as regularity of bowel movement, of sleeping time, and of other manifestations of our biological rhythm—depend on habits.

We use drugs occasionally, but food daily; the need for a good eating habit becomes vital. Thoughtless departures from a good eating habit can create problems and adversely affect our health. This means that falling in line with every new food craze is unwise—at least. But it also means that though nutrition has certain basic beliefs that are presently considered good, they may be found to be faulty when new findings disclose more information. Therefore, while we cannot fall for every new nutritional craze neither can we afford to be dogmatic.

How do you keep to the narrow line between nutritional anarchy and nutritional rigidity?

It is not easy. It requires more than information—judgment based upon adequate knowledge is necessary.

Nutrition is a highly complex process. It is also loaded with ambiguities because people often use words for what they want them to mean. When people speak of a "healthy diet" they may be referring to the particular nutritional dogma they practice. When a physician advises a patient to eat a "good diet" it can be equally meaningless unless qualified: what is a good diet in terms of the patient's condition? More likely than not, the patient has some problems and in fact that is the reason he went to see his physician. Is a so-called good diet the same for him as for a person without that particular problem? It may not be, or we may not know. How often when someone evangelizes in behalf of a high potassium intake in the diet, does he realize that, while potassium is an essential element, it is virtually poison to an individual with disease of the adrenals (such as Addison's disease) and to some people with heart disease?

This book is not about nutrition but is an assessment of the role of vitamin E in nutrition. However, several definitions relating to nutrition may be helpful to the reader:

(1) Nutrition is the process of assimilating food for the purposes of providing and sustaining energy, promoting growth, and replacing normal tissue loss.

(2) Nourishment is food or a material that provides nutrition.

(3) A nutrient is something that provides nourishment; the term may also be used as an adjective, for example, nutrient substance. A secondary nutrient (for instance, lactose) is something that stimulates the intestinal microorganisms to produce other nutrients.

(4) A diet is a list of substances to be consumed per day or other period of time. A diet usually is inclusive (that is, what should be eaten) as well as exclusive (that is, what to avoid). A "good diet" is intended to make an animal grow, mature, and reproduce.

This definition of a good diet fits all animals with some exceptions. For example, a rat can have adequate growth and otherwise adequate health but still have some pathological conditions due to vitamin E deficiency. Another exception to this definition applies in the case of man, who in addition needs a healthy psychological input to mature. An obvious exception to this definition is in the case of women past the childbearing age in whom reproduction is not possible.

We should have a better definition of diet. Although standard diets are reasonably suitable for most people most of the time, they do not fulfill special requirements for periods of stress—such as illness, pregnancy, adolescence, old age. With this recognition in mind, we should usually modify our standard diet in stressful periods by inclusion as well as exclusion to provide optimal nourishment—provided we know what optimal nourishment is in the specific case.

A balanced diet is one that contains all the necessary factors for good nourishment: proteins, carbohydrates, fats, vitamins, and minerals. But even this definition is faulty when quantities are not set forth for the special purpose that a diet is to fulfill. For example, a diet which contains just 2 grams of protein per day theoretically is balanced. In effect, it is not balanced because 2 grams of protein a day is not enough for anyone.

Various diets.

Diets are subject to considerable controversy and a great deal of personal eccentricity.

The following types of diet are frequently recommended—often with poor judgment:

Alkaline ash diet: A basic, or alkaline ash, diet is one that consists largely of fruits, some milk, and vegetables. The word "basic" has nothing to do with "fundamental"—it refers to a base, namely an alkali.

Acid ash diet: Conversely, an acid ash diet is one which consists largely of high protein foods, namely fish, meat, eggs, and also cereals, including breads.

Dissociated diet: A dissociated diet is one in which proteins are eaten at one meal and carbohydrates at another. Its fad value was high at one time.

Ketogenic diet: A ketogenic diet is one consisting largely of fat—with only small amounts of proteins and carbohydrates. When fat breaks down it produces fatty acids and certain ketones. There are occasional medical reasons for which this diet is recommended but it should not be used unless so directed by a physician—for good reason.

Aside from the foods which provide proteins, carbohydrates, and fats, the normal diet must contain other elements, namely water and accessory food substances. These substances are the vitamins; if there is a deficiency in vitamins, disease conditions set in. And the diet also requires certain metals—such as copper, manganese, cobalt, etc.—in minute amounts. These are referred to as trace minerals, or trace metals, because their presence in traces is often sufficient. Sodium, magnesium, potassium, iron, and calcium are also metals, but larger amounts are required—much more than traces. These "macro-metals" are usually supplied in food, except if there are certain restrictions in the diet—such as the deficiency of calcium in a milk-free diet, or the deficiency of iron in a largely milk diet.

The American diet.

We often hear that all the American public needs in vitamins—and usually trace metals—is supplied in the American grocery basket, that is, in the foods normally eaten. This is the party line, which unfortunately has been too often heard. Outstanding nutritionists—such as Dr. Roger J. Williams, director of the Clayton Foundation Biochemical Institute of the University of Texas at Austin, a creative scientist and the discoverer of pantothenic acid and other B vitamins—have often deplored it.

Ample quantities of vitamins and minerals may well be found in food, but one cannot depend on food alone for them for several reasons:

(1) The method of food preparation often causes deterioration of certain vitamins—they may be oxidized by heat or leached out in the cooking water, which is then thrown out.

(2) People have a variety of personal dislikes and usually do not choose to eat the foods they dislike. Thus, the American diet—or any other diet—becomes skewed.

(3) Ethnic considerations often work against a consumer receiving all the vitamins or minerals that are purportedly present in the regular American diet, simply because certain ethnic groups do not eat many of the common American foods. For example, the increasing Puerto Rican population in New York holds to its own dietary habits. In addition, even a substance as American as hominy grits leaves much to be desired, if the grits are a considerable quantitative factor in the diet, because grits are virtually all carbohydrate.

(4) Storage as well as commercial processing of food

reduces the vitamin content—this is particularly true of vitamin E.

(5) Economic considerations often preclude buying foods which constitute the so-called regular American diet: this is true of people in poverty pockets, of old people who live on social security with its minimal dole or on a small pension, and especially of those on welfare. In fact, such people do not have enough money to buy an adequate variety of food, let alone supplementary vitamins.

(6) Dietary preferences among people, especially old people who hold stubbornly to certain dietary exclusions based on old customs or capriciousness, sometimes prevent them from receiving all the good which is inherent in the regular American diet. Dietary preferences among the young may have the same effect—some of them, especially teen-age girls who want to conform to their ideal of a figure, often exist but cannot thrive on a diet of coffee, orange juice, and cola drinks.

(7) Geographical differences—especially in vegetables—prevent reliance on a stable amount of vitamins and minerals in the so-called regular American diet.

(8) What is the regular American diet? Is there such a thing? Except in broad generalities, regional differences in dietary habits prevent us from believing that there is a standard American diet consumed everywhere in the 50 states. Remember that it was only about a generation ago that reliance on the regular American diet in the South produced pellagra. There is no danger of pellagra now because of the enrichment of food with vitamins that has almost wiped out pellagra. And even though enriched bread (enriched by nicotinic acid) prevents pellagra, people who eat potatoes or rice instead obviously cannot have the benefit of enrichment.

(9) Seasonal variations prevent reliance on certain vitamins. For example, the vitamin E in cow's milk varies from 0.2 milligram per quart in the early spring to 1.6 milligrams per quart in the fall—an eightfold difference.

(10) The average American diet according to various investigators probably supplies only 7 milligrams of α-tocopherol a day, which is far from enough. Storage, freezing, frying, and other commercial food-processing operations further reduce the vitamin E level.

For some reason, the subject of nutrition is fraught with a good deal of passion. It results in evangelistic fervor on the one hand, and in rigid resistance or polemics on the other.

If we define learning as a constructive change in behavior resulting from previous experience, most of us do not learn easily. This refers to the faddist who sees the world in terms of vitamins as well as to the person who hews close to the establishmentarian contention that the American grocery basket has all the vitamins and minerals we need.

That type of zeal versus resistance is especially true of vitamins.

Lack of vitamin A.

Let us consider one vitamin—namely vitamin A, against which, unlike vitamin E, there is really no serious resistance. Perhaps in this case we may have learned a little, but we will not have learned if we depend solely on food to supply all our vitamins.

For example: during the Third Western Hemisphere Nutrition Congress, held in the summer of 1971, of which the American Medical Association and the American Institute of Nutrition were two of the sponsors and organizers, Dr. T. K. Murray, chief of the

Nutrition Research Division of Canada's Food and Drug Directorate, said that:

> Low intakes and even low vitamin A blood levels have been found with no physical symptoms apparent. But in at least one survey, among children of migrant workers in Colorado, investigators found significant correlations between low vitamin A levels and the incidence of skin and upper respiratory infections and several other symptoms.

He also reported that:

> A significant percentage of most age groups in North America lack appreciable liver reserves of vitamin A, and 20% to 30% fail to consume the recommended daily allowance. And although most North American adults have adequate blood levels of vitamin A, an important number of children fall below the acceptable level, with adverse health effects to some of them.

To help solve the problem he recommended further study toward better defining human needs, care in replacing vitamin A lost during processing of foods, and addition of vitamin A to some basic foods such as flour.

Dr. Murray's comments hit the mark—and remind us that we must not lose sight of our objectives, and that we ought not to wait until a deficiency is reached before we sound an alarm as to vitamin intake: "Let us not argue about the fine details of the problem with such fervor that we forget the goal—an acceptable vitamin A status for the whole population."

These are the problems found with vitamin A—a fully "accepted" vitamin.

Can you imagine what problems and resistances occur with vitamin E?

Need for vitamin E.

After long resistance, vitamin E is now considered essential to the body economy by the Food and Drug Administration. Only the amount has not been legally fixed and frozen into Minimum Daily Requirement provisions. This is what is meant by the phrase "minimum daily requirement not established."

In the meantime, the prestigious Food and Nutrition Board of the National Academy of Sciences and National Research Council recognized in 1964 that vitamin E is essential for man and published in 1968 the Recommended Dietary Allowances—the daily amounts of vitamin E required by the following groups of people:

Infants	0-1 year	5 I.U.
Children	1-6 years	10 I.U.
Children	6-10 years	15 I.U.
Children	10-14 years	20 I.U.
Males	14-18 years	25 I.U.
Males	18-75 years	30 I.U.
Females	14-75 years	25 I.U.
Lactating and Pregnant Women		30 I.U.

These are only guiding figures—the daily amounts needed are probably appreciably larger. For example, the more polyunsaturated fatty acids in the diet, the greater the amount of vitamin E that is necessary.

Vitamin E is formed only in plants and is not produced by animals or man in the body as some vitamins are. It can be obtained from the diet, but supplementary amounts are probably needed for a number of reasons, one of which has to do with the amount of polyunsaturated fatty acids a person consumes in food. Vitamin E is stored in the body—more specifically in the liver and fatty tissue—which possibly accounts for the absence of dramatic deficiency symptoms for a long time. Though about 7% of people, according to some investigators, are deficient in vitamin E as deduced from low vitamin E levels in the blood, there is no unanimity on specifically how much vitamin E is necessary.

Many plants and plant substances—such as green lettuce, peanuts, wheat germ, and cottonseed, corn, and safflower oils—as well as meat, butter, eggs, and fish liver oils normally contain vitamin E or tocopherols. The vitamin E preserves the oils from rancidity, which is a manifestation of oxidation.

But other plant oils, such as olive oil and coconut oil, that do not contain tocopherols do not oxidize readily. What saves them from oxidation is their *saturated* bonds—they are *not* unsaturated. Only unsaturated compounds have extra places on their molecules, which offer a home for oxygen—hence oxidation. And vitamin E is contained only in unsaturated oils.

The more oils containing polyunsaturated fatty acids consumed in the diet, the greater the nutritional need for vitamin E. The reason for this lies in the fact that polyunsaturated fatty acids need extra vitamin E to retain their unsaturation and take it from the vitamin E in the body—thus making the body's reserve of vitamin E unavailable for its antioxidant purposes to the body economy as a whole. That is the reason why polyunsaturated fatty acids increase the need for vitamin E.

Vitamin E is a fat soluble vitamin, but it can be utilized by the body even though the diet is extremely low in fat, as long as it is taken supplementally and there is no malabsorption, which prevents its utilization.

The large number and diversity of biochemical processes that go on in the body in connection with the utilization of food are almost inconceivable. While we may conceive their enormity, we do not fully understand the interrelationships of the processes. By processes we mean the transactions of enzymes: the enzyme itself; the material on which it acts (called the substrate); the resulting substance or substances; and the feedback of the resulting substances into the first reaction of enzyme and substrate. The rate of the reactions is always influenced by the buildup of the resulting substance, which often acts as a governor by limiting the rate of reaction after a given buildup. Scores of other events are initiated when an enzyme acts upon a substrate.

All these events go on in connection with one enzyme. Multiply by the numbers of enzymes and add exponential power to the interplay of dozens of enzymes, each taking place simultaneously in one vessel—the body—and you will surely find that the number of processes must surpass the number of stars in the sky.

Enzymes both act upon other substances and are acted upon. Two of the most frequent reactions among enzymes are oxidation and reduction. They work in tandem: when something is oxidized, something else is reduced. When only one step is interrupted, a dozen or more steps may stop or may act in ways that can be abnormal.

Consider the role of an antioxidant in such a welter of activity. If there is nothing to check oxidation, it may proceed wildly and create the sort of damage discussed in previous paragraphs. There is a natural tendency to oxidation, hence the need for an antioxidant. Conversely, there is also a need for oxidation in many life processes.

This is the reason for the importance of vitamin E, an antioxidant. At least, this is a partial reason because the role of vitamin E is far from well understood. The above paragraphs are a schematic explanation, an oversimplified view, but hopefully show a small but important part of the role played by vitamin E.

Amount.

As far as is now known, only a comparatively small amount of vitamin E is necessary to be useful. But our knowledge is imperfect because of the presence of other variables, many of which are also unknown or uncertain. Only 0.5 milligram of vitamin E per 100 milliliters of blood is necessary—below this level deficiency in vitamin E sets in. Half a milligram is equivalent to about 1/120 of a grain—in terms of pinheads, perhaps half a pinhead—while 100 milliliters (or cc) are equivalent to about 3⅓ fluid ounces.

The amount of vitamin E necessary in the daily diet was said to be dependent upon the amount of polyunsaturated fatty acids in the diet—the more polyunsaturated fatty acids, the more vitamin E needed. The specific polyunsaturated fatty acids in the diet are linoleic acid and arachidonic acid—along with lesser unsaturated fatty acids. (The chapter on foods gives further details as to unsaturated fatty acid contents of various food substances.) The requirement commonly considered adequate to prevent deficiency is 30 milligrams a day, as set by the guidelines of the Recommended Daily Allowance of the Food and Nutrition Board of the National Academy of Sciences and National Research Council. If taken in the form of tablets or capsules, 100 I.U. daily should probably be adequate to allow for the variety of functions of vitamin E. Considerably more is often taken, and one cannot meaningfully speak of an average dose. But when we speak of amounts of vitamin E necessary in the daily diet, we must consider another variable. That is, when the unsaturated fatty acids have been oxidized, larger amounts of vitamin E become necessary both to prevent further oxidation and to *hope* to create a reversal.

But a note about the small quantity of vitamin E needed: some vitamins—and in fact most trace minerals—act as catalytic agents; that is, they initiate or hasten a reaction but are themselves not consumed. For that reason extremely small quantities are needed.

But vitamin E is itself consumed in part in the process of blocking oxidation—it acts sacrificially by allowing oxidation to take place on itself, thus robbing oxidizing agents of their power to damage tissue components. This is yet another variable. In the absence of more knowledge, it is more logical to make more vitamin E available to the body rather than less, especially in light of the fact that no toxic effects have been reported.

These are a few of the variables about which something is known. The variables we do not know about cannot be assessed and perhaps may turn out to be more important. In fact, Dr. M. K. Horwitt hypothesizes that chronic disease may well be due to vitamin E deprivation.

The effects of vitamin E deficiency have been considered in other chapters (on malabsorption, on polyunsaturated fatty acids, etc.) in their different contexts.

Malnutrition.

Nutrition suggests its opposite condition: malnutrition. Unfortunately, malnutrition is often understood to be the condition in which there is not enough to eat. It is considered synonymous with hunger—*which it is not.* Malnutrition is exactly that which is implied by its name: *mal,* or bad, nutrition. One can even have an overabundant diet, grow overweight from it, and be malnourished. Malnutrition can occur, for example, when an overabundance of starches and fats but too little protein is consumed, as in certain ethnic diets. Malnutrition can also set in when there is a deficiency of the accessory food substances—vitamins and minerals.

While this book is about vitamin E, it does not advocate vitamin E—or anything else for that matter. For that reason it is emphasized that the accessory foods intake should include the vitamins and minerals known to be essential, as well as those considered at this time to be unessential. We make the last point—which is an unpopular one—because the essentiality of a vitamin or other food substance is often a legal definition rather than a scientific finding. You do not need facts for an edict—but you need them, among other needs, for a scientific truth.

For example, remember that *less than 10 years ago vitamin E was considered unessential.* Animals then growing that were not exposed to vitamin E may have been harmed.

An insidious form of malnutrition is borderline malnutrition. Frank symptoms of malnutrition are easily recognized. Symptoms of borderline malnutrition are usually ascribed to other causes—it is easier to do so than to get out on a limb.

Borderline malnutrition may be caused by the following conditions:

Pressures from peers: Bizarre eating habits that follow peer pressures rather than nutritional wisdom can produce borderline malnutrition. For example, the attempt by adolescents to handle acne sets up such fads as avoiding milk.

Mental fog: Produced by long-standing borderline or actual malnutrition, mental fog is not blamed upon idiotic food habits but often on Democrats, Republicans, the New Left or the Old Reactionaries, meat, corn, or hormones in beef. Examples of bizarre diets, the long-term effects of some of which we do not yet know, are meatless diets for growing people, macrobiotic and other crank diets that are more mystically than nutritionally oriented, raw food fads, etc. These diversions are usually practiced not by a lunatic fringe but by "normal" and prudent people who merely exaggerate an idea until it becomes a caricature—an example is the swing from justifiable protests against war to avoidance of killing of food animals, hence avoidance of meat and fish. Dr. George M. Briggs, professor of nutrition at the University of California at Berkeley, estimates that half a million people in California have ceased to eat meat.

Dental and social conditions: Dentures may make chewing unpleasant; hence people troubled with poorly fitting dentures may avoid foods that may be nutritionally desirable. Also, recluses often live on toast and tea or on potatoes, bread, and jam. Such diets produce borderline malnutrition that leads to mental deterioration (which is ascribed to senility rather than to nutritional inadequacy). Many older people cannot afford to buy the vitamins necessary to supplement their dangerous diet.

Illness: Fever, colds, or immobility due to fractures may lead to loss of appetite and borderline malnutrition. Other stresses, such as hyperthyroidism, increase metabolism and the need for vitamins B_1 and C, among other vitamins. Malabsorption clearly demands assurance that the foodstuffs and vitamins ingested are absorbed. In malabsorption there is a definite bar to the absorption of the fat-soluble vitamins—A, D, E, and K—and a reduced absorption of the water-soluble vitamins, minerals, and water.

Ignorance of nutrition.

What we know about nutrition is comparatively little—about vitamin E we know less. Even in such a well-known vitamin as vitamin C, new work continues to disclose that its role may be much more than simply that of a water-soluble antioxidant. For example, Dr. E. M. Baker III and his associates, of the U. S. Army Medical Research and Nutrition Laboratory of Denver's Fitzsimmons General Hospital, studied the excretion products of vitamin C and found a number of hitherto unknown derivatives in the urine. Finding hitherto unknown derivatives suggests that hitherto unknown functions of vitamin C exist in man. The reason is that different functions have different excretion products.

Nutrition is more than food and feeding with its direct result on health. It has far-reaching sociological importance, changing the population in rural and urban communities and making city slums worse.

This belief is based on the finding that poor families in rural communities eat worse than those in the city, as concluded by Dr. Carlos L. Krumdiek of the departments of medicine and pediatrics of the University of Alabama Medical Center in Birmingham. Dr. Krumdiek states in the March 8, 1971, issue of the *Journal of the American Medical Association* that "rural malnutrition is the only one factor which seems to be common to all cases of rural to urban migrations throughout the world."

The reason for this state of affairs is that farmers now produce one or two cash crops and buy their food in the grocery store, while in the past the farm family grew most of its own food in addition to producing cash crops.

Does it sound incredible that despite the expenditure of billions of dollars in government funds for medical research, there is a widespread ignorance of nutrition, even among scientists? Have you wondered why, throughout this book, you find numerous statements that such-and-such is not known, or that it *possibly* may be thus-and-so, but there is no generally accepted consensus among scientists for the explanation of a given phenomenon?

Dr. Roger J. Williams, the biochemist to whom we previously referred, gives what he believes is a reason for our poor state of knowledge of nutrition and for our relative ignorance of the relation between nutrition and health. He reminds us that there is no institution anywhere in the world which studies any disease from the standpoint of the role that nutrition may play in its development and its conversion to chronic disease. He refers to degenerative diseases, such as arthritis and atherosclerosis, and other serious diseases, such as mental diseases, which can hit at any age.

Funds for the study of diseases depend largely on two factors: emotional and political pressures. Poliomyelitis was conquered because of the emotional pressure generated by the public, which was touched by pictures of polio children in braces. Cancer is another special disease—it is sensitive to political pressure. What politician will risk his political neck by voting *for* cancer, by withholding funds. Both diseases—though serious indeed—carry forth strong emotional reactions and hence public pressure.

Nutrition and disease.

But nutrition? It does not have the emotional appeal, though it can well be the most important study in the *prevention* of numerous diseases. Through the daily practice of poor nutrition, a solid groundwork is laid for the slow development of diseases that, by their slow development, have their chronic nature embedded. Poor nutrition reduces our natural resistance to disease —the first line of defense against any disease. Dr. M. K. Horwitt, who was previously mentioned, may indeed be right in stating that vitamin E deprivation may be the reason for the chronicity of disease. We would modify that to state that such deprivation may well be one of the important reasons.

Natural resistance would take many pages to define accurately—if in fact, it can be defined. Remember that our understanding of what constitutes natural resistance has many areas of ignorance.

But natural resistance can be epitomized by considering one illustration: doctors concerned with venereal disease often see in their case findings the phenomenon of a man who develops gonorrhea from sexual contact with a given women, while another man who has had sexual relations with the same woman at about the same time may not develop it. This phenomenon is ascribed to a difference in natural resistance—because we do not understand the precise cause for such a happening.

Most recently, in an article in the respected research journal *Perspectives in Biology and Medicine,* Dr. Roger J. Williams pleads for a serious concern in teaching of clinical nutrition by the nation's medical schools. That topic is largely neglected, except for teaching the basic biochemistry and physiology. A fine professional journal, the *American Journal of Clinical Nutrition,* does exist. But nutrition, through default by the medical schools, has largely fallen into the hands of many faddists—though knowledgeable people exist among them. And in all fairness it must be said that in some instances they were prophetic—they turned out to be right in their push to less-processed foods, for instance.

When your doctor tells you to eat a "good diet," it may have no meaning for you, and it may well not have for him. But do not blame him. Nutrition, though basic and vital to life, does not have the emotional appeal that, for example, polio has and therefore suffers from neglect of attention and appropriations of time and money.

Cholesterol.

The question whether the cholesterol-rich American diet is substantially responsible for hardening of the arteries is not yet resolved. For example, the world-renowned Dr. Irvine H. Page, consultant-emeritus of the Cleveland Clinic, holds that it is not cholesterol per se that should be blamed for the incidence of heart disease in the U.S.A. but a combination of many factors, among which are stress, smoking, obesity, exercise, and genetics as well as dietary factors. Dr. Page has been for years in the forefront of research on heart disease in the United States.

On the other hand, at a meeting of the American Heart Association during the fall of 1971, at Anaheim, California, Dr. Robert Wissler, of the University of Chicago, supported the idea that the American diet does go a long way in producing arteriosclerosis. In his experiments, rhesus monkeys (which have many nutritional similarities to man) in just two years developed hardening of the arteries, or arteriosclerosis, on the "typical American diet" with its higher fats, cholesterol, and refined sugar. Their hardening of the arteries was four times as severe as that of a group of monkeys on a diet lower in fats, cholesterol, and refined sugar.

Is there a doubt that much more research in nutrition is needed?

We have many roadmarkers but relatively few conclusive cornerstones in nutrition. It is still a science-in-the-making; hence we cannot afford to discard, out-of-hand, any subjective information upon which it hits. Again, Albert Einstein said it most poignantly and pointedly:

Science Existing is the most logically consistent discipline known to man. Science-in-the-Making on the other hand, is as subjective and as psychologically conditioned as any branch of human endeavor.

CHAPTER 11

Trace Metals

Trace metals (also trace minerals or trace elements) are so named because they occur in minute amounts, that is, in *traces,* largely in plants, in rocks of the earth's crust, and in animals. Some trace metals appear to be necessary or even critical in a variety of biochemical happenings that take place in metabolism. Some trace metals may have more than one function. One example of a trace metal is copper—which is necessary as a catalyst in the utilization of iron by the body in blood-building.

The giant studies in trace metals were done by Dr. Henry A. Schroeder, Emeritus Professor of Physiology in the Dartmouth Medical School, who virtually opened this field when it was little more than a curiosity. There are other investigators, especially in foreign countries. The contributions of Dr. Schroeder and his coworkers, Drs. Balassa, Gibson, Valanju, Hogencamp, and Tipton have included studies on the toxicity, role, and need of most trace metals—including manganese, cadmium, chromium, vanadium, zinc, nickel, lead, titanium, cobalt, copper, molybdenum, and selenium.

The role of many trace metals in nutrition is not clear—the role of others is extremely important. Some trace metals, such as aluminum, antimony, fluorine, arsenic, barium, cadmium, and chromium, have been found to occur *in minute quantities* in body organs of certain animals. If they have a function it is unknown. They may possibly function as catalysts to regulate the metabolism of enzymes.

Some trace metals interact with others or are necessary to the function of other metals. The interaction between copper and iron is an example. Copper aids in the utilization of iron. Hemoglobin contains both iron and copper.

Other trace metals are clearly toxic—such as barium or cadmium. There is no known use for cadmium in the animal body economy.

Cobalt.

Cobalt, a metal, is part of vitamin B_{12}. A very small quantity—0.1 microgram (there are 1,000 micrograms to a milligram and 1,000 milligrams to a gram, and about 28 grams to an ounce)—a day is needed to synthesize enough vitamin B_{12}. It is calculated that the "normal" diet supplies probably 5 micrograms a day. While cobalt is necessary to blood building, too much of the good thing is dangerous. Excessive amounts may cause, in some animals, a condition called polycythemia in which there is a huge increase of red blood cells, which in turn interferes with oxygen metabolism. An overload in the body can be caused by other metals or minerals such as iron. While iron is necessary, an excessive amount of iron causes iron storage disease, which also interferes with other functions in body metabolism.

Magnesium.

Magnesium, although not strictly a trace metal because more than traces are concerned, is another metal necessary in the body function. It is calculated that through the average daily diet about 300 milligrams are taken per day. Magnesium is involved in perhaps a greater number of physiologic functions than other metals. Magnesium activates the function of adenosine triphosphate (ATP), which is a key in energy metabolism. It is involved also in muscle contraction, in carbohydrate and fat metabolism, and in the utilization of certain B vitamins (thiamine pyrophosphate). When there is a deficiency of magnesium some of the signs are similar to calcium deficiency, that is, the production of tetany or spasm.

As a matter of fact, there is an interrelationship between magnesium and calcium. For example, in a diet low in phosphorus, an excessive amount of magnesium will stimulate a loss of calcium in the body. This is stopped when phosphorus is added. Conversely, excess of calcium can produce a deficiency of magnesium.

Zinc.

Zinc is an important metal, because it is a component of certain enzyme systems. It is calculated that the average diet supplies probably 10 to 15 milligrams per day. Zinc accumulates in virtually all tissues and has specific functions in certain organs, such as the pancreas, muscles, and prostate and in red blood cells.

How is this related to vitamin E? Probably, not at all.

However, the above picture of trace metals is presented to offer a framework to the reader, since one trace metal, selenium, does have an important relationship to vitamin E.

Selenium and vitamin E.

But do not take selenium. It is an extremely poisonous metal. Selenium is related to vitamin E simply because it has *some* of the properties of vitamin E, but not others. About two decades ago it became known that a minute quantity of selenium—one part selenium in *ten million* parts of chicken feed—overcame some of the effects of vitamin E deprivation in chicks.

One of the great researchers in vitamin E, Dr. A. L. Tappel, also reported that the same proportion of selenium—one part in ten million—was able to substitute for vitamin E in *some* animals for *some* conditions. What probably happens is that selenium acts as a fat antioxidant, much the same as vitamin E. But that is not the complete story.

Selenium is extremely toxic for all animals as well as for man. A proportion of only ten parts per million can kill. Occasionally pasture lands relatively high in selenium have killed herds of cattle and sheep that have eaten the vegetation growing on these lands.

Selenium is present in probably a smaller quantity in the earth's crust than all but a few elements—only 0.09 part per million, or less than one part in ten million. It is present in sea water in even a smaller amount—about 1/20 as much.

Some of the effects of selenium—but in minute quantities—are similar to those of vitamin E in animals. Selenium prevents muscular dystrophy in poults, exudative diathesis in chicks, white muscle disease in cattle and sheep. Some animals probably require selenium even though they may be given vitamin E.

It is fascinating to consider that the role of selenium in preventing liver necrosis in animals was found only when it was realized that selenium was a contaminant in two sulfur-containing amino acids, methionine and cystine, that were administered. When these amino acids were purified so that they did not have a trace of selenium they no longer prevented liver necrosis!

Various opinions exist on the question whether selenium is an essential dietary substance in its own right or if by sparing vitamin E, it potentiates it. One view is that like vitamin E, selenium acts as a free-radical immobilizer, or scavenger. It is indeed important in animal feed, but its role in man, though it is considered essential by some, is far from proved.

Minute and varying quantities of selenium occur naturally in seafood, tuna, anchovies, herring, menhaden, brewer's yeast, wheat germ, bran, broccoli, cabbage, tomato, meat, and grains. The richest natural sources of selenium are shrimp, lobster, smelt, fish flour, smoked herring filets, pork kidney, beef kidney, and Brazil nuts.

Selenium is a highly toxic material. If you take vitamin E *do not try to spike it with selenium—it can kill.* But there is no objection to eating foods containing selenium as described above, provided that they are not taken in excess in order to build up selenium reserves. They can tear down too.

The immense number of variables as to the reciprocal- and counter-reactions involved in the relation between trace metals and the functioning of the body make a reliable understanding of their role difficult. These are not new problems. Recognized even by the ancient Romans, the point was well summed up by Horace, who was born about 65 B.C.:

> The very difficulty of a problem evokes abilities or talents which would otherwise, in happy times, never emerge to shine.

CHAPTER 12

Vitamin E in Foods

Various foods contain vitamin E. To choose the one that contains the highest amount of vitamin E is often a mistake!

Why?

Because while several tocopherols—alpha-, beta-, and gamma-tocopherols are all "vitamin E" (see Chapter 1)—only *alpha-tocopherol* is the variant that has the highest biological activity. This is especially important when assessing foods for vitamin E content, because most foods, unlike tablets or capsules of vitamin E, are not labeled with their alpha-tocopherol equivalents. However, many prepared or canned foods are so labeled.

The question to be resolved is what proportion of *alpha*-tocopherol a given food contains. For example, about 90% of the tocopherol in safflower oil is alpha-tocopherol. But only 20% of the tocopherol in corn or soybean oil is alpha-tocopherol. This does not mean that corn oil should not be used—there are other reasons for using it. But it does mean that one should be

ALPHA-TOCOPHEROL CONTENT OF FOODS*

Vitamin E Content of Foods

Product	Total Tocopherol (mg. %)	α-Tocopherol (mg. %)	% Lipid	α-Tocopherol (mg./gm. Lipid)
MEATS				
Bacon (fried)	0.59	0.53	39.7	0.001
Ham steak (fried)	0.52	0.28	6.8	0.04
Pork sausage (fried)	0.32	0.16	35.0	0.005
Liverwurst	0.69	0.35	27.0	0.013
Bologna	0.49	0.06	26.6	0.002
Salami	0.68	0.11	16.0	0.007
Ground beef (pan fried)	0.63	0.37	11.1	0.033
Fresh beef liver (broiled)	1.62	0.63	5.8	0.11
Fresh veal cutlet (pan fried)	0.24	0.05	1.6	0.03
T bone beef steak (broiled)	0.55	0.13	9.5	0.014
Lamb chops (broiled)	0.32	0.16	13.3	0.012
Pork chops (pan fried)	0.60	0.16	19.5	0.008
FISH				
Fillet of haddock (broiled)	1.20	0.60	0.18	3.3
Salmon steak (broiled)	1.81	1.35	3.20	0.42
Deep fried frozen shrimp				
Oven heated	6.6	0.6	12.9	0.047
Not heated	5.9	1.9	11.5	0.165
Deep fried frozen scallops				
Oven heated	6.2	0.60	9.4	0.064
Not heated	3.9	0.71	5.9	0.12
POULTRY				
Chicken breast (broiled)	0.58	0.37	3.90	0.095
Frozen fried chicken				
Brand "A"				
Oven heated	0.32	0.04	23.8	0.002
Brand "A-1"*				
Oven heated	1.39	0.38	20.0	0.019
Not heated	1.43	0.40	19.0	0.021
Brand "B"				
Oven heated	1.10	0.16	18.0	0.009
Not heated	0.80	0.10	14.0	0.007
VEGETABLES				
Raw potato	0.085	0.053	—	—
Baked potato	0.055	0.027	—	—
Boiled potato	0.061	0.043	—	—
Frozen french fried potatoes				
Brand "A"**				
Oven heated	0.36	0.12	6.8	0.018
Not heated	0.64	0.15	5.5	0.027
Brand "B"				
Oven heated	1.59	0.43	6.2	0.069
Not heated	1.22	0.41	5.4	0.076
Fresh yellow onion	0.34	0.22	—	—
Frozen french fried onion rings				
Brand "A"				
Oven heated	6.2	0.72	25.6	0.028
Not heated	5.2	0.60	20.6	0.029

*Reproduced by the permission of The American Journal of Clinical Nutrition, Vol. 17, No. 1, 1965.

**Same as "A" but bought at a different store.

Product	Total Tocopherol (mg. %)	α-Tocopherol (mg. %)	% Lipid	α-Tocopherol (mg./gm. Lipid)
Brand "B"				
Oven heated	6.4	0.65	23.2	0.028
Not heated	5.5	0.52	17.2	0.030
Baked beans, Boston style	1.16	0.14	—	—
Fresh peas	1.73	0.55	1.74	0.32
Canned green peas	0.04	0.02	—	—
Frozen green peas				
Cooked	0.65	0.25	—	—
Uncooked	0.64	0.22	—	—
Canned green beans	0.05	0.03	—	—
Frozen cut green beans				
Cooked	0.25	0.11	—	—
Uncooked	0.24	0.09	—	—
Canned leaf spinach	0.06	0.02	—	—
Canned kernel corn	0.09	0,05	—	—
Frozen kernel corn				
Cooked	0.48	0.19	—	—
Uncooked	0.49	0.19	—	—
Celery	0.57	0.38	0.116	3.3
Carrots	0.21	0.11	0.046	2.4
Lettuce	0.17	0.061	0.112	0.55
Fresh tomatoes	0.85	0.40	0.074	5.4
Dry navy beans	1.68	0.47	0.60	0.78
Cooked white rice	0.27	0.18	0.50	0.36

FRUITS AND FRUIT JUICES

Product	Total Tocopherol (mg. %)	α-Tocopherol (mg. %)	% Lipid	α-Tocopherol (mg./gm. Lipid)
Fresh strawberries	0.29	0.13	0.128	1.02
Frozen sliced strawberries	0.40	0.21	0.069	3.04
Fresh banana	0.42	0.22	0.29	0.76
Fresh cantaloupe melon	0.31	0.14	0.20	0.70
Fresh apple	0.51	0.31	0.19	1.63
Canned tomato juice	0.71	0.22	—	—
Canned grapefruit juice	0.18	0.04	—	—
Fresh orange juice	0.20	0.04	—	—

BREADS

Product	Total Tocopherol (mg. %)	α-Tocopherol (mg. %)	% Lipid	α-Tocopherol (mg./gm. Lipid)
White bread	0.23	0.10	2.6	0.05
Whole wheat bread	2.2	0.45	2.8	0.16

CEREALS

Product	Total Tocopherol (mg. %)	α-Tocopherol (mg. %)	% Lipid	α-Tocopherol (mg./gm. Lipid)
Oatmeal	3.23	2.27	6.33	0.36
Corn flakes	0.43	0.12	0.33	0.36
Dry processed rice cereal	0.28	0.04	0.2	0.2
Dry oat cereal	1.53	0.60	2.3	0.26
Yellow corn meal	3.43	0.64	3.80	0.17
Hominy grits	1.17	0.31	0.9	0.34
Processed wheat and barley cereal	2.45	0.61	0.98	0.62

Product	Total Tocopherol (mg. %)	α-Tocopherol (mg. %)	% Lipid	α-Tocopherol (mg./gm. Lipid)
DESSERTS				
Chocolate ice cream				
Brand "A"	1.02	0.36	12.2	0.03
Brand "B"	1.10	0.37	10.7	0.035
Vanilla ice cream	0.39	0.06	13.2	0.005
Fresh baked apple pie	15.7	2.50	10.6	0.24
Fresh baked blueberry pie	17.7	3.12	14.7	0.21
Fresh pound cake	7.4	1.1	22.0	0.05
Chocolate cupcake	2.0	0.14	17.2	0.008
Milk chocolate bar	4.2	1.1	29.8	0.037
Peanut butter/oatmeal cookie	7.67	6.0	24.0	0.25
Shortbread cookie	1.33	0.46	24.7	0.02
Wafer type cookie	1.43	0.53	10.8	0.05
Chocolate/cream cookie	2.81	1.29	17.5	0.07
MISCELLANEOUS				
Mustard	4.15	1.75	3.50	0.50
Whole milk	0.093	0.036	3.40	0.011
Butter	1.0	1.0	----	----
Egg	1.43	0.46	7.0	0.066
Corn oil margarine, brand "A"	46.7	13.2	80.0	0.17
Soya and cottonseed oils margarine, brand "B"	59.5	13.0	82.0	0.16
Cocktail peanuts	11.2	6.7	50.3	0.13
Dry roasted peanuts	11.7	7.7	49.3	0.15
Instant coffee	0.48	nil		
Cottonseed oil mayonnaise, brand "A"	9.0	6.0	11.0	0.54
Mayonnaise, brand "B"	50.0	24.3	66.0	0.37
Polyunsaturated mayonnaise, brand "C"	42.0	8.6	76.4	0.11
Potato chips	11.4	6.4	44.8	0.14
Pretzel sticks	0.77	0.15	1.62	0.09
Club cracker	1.17	0.80	16.6	0.05

aware of the facts in order to have a proper view of vitamin E, or alpha-tocopherol, contents in various foods.

When you look for vitamin E content in food, also determine if the vitamin E content applies to the food as it is bought, or after preparation. For example, the average loss of vitamin E after processing or cooking ranges from 35% to 90% in corn, wheat, oats, and rice. The loss of vitamin E in samples selected for assay by scientists Drs. Herting and Drury, researchers in vitamin E, ranged from 35% in white corn meal to 98% for corn flakes; other losses in processing wheat ranged from 22% to 92%. In rice cereal products the loss in vitamin E during production was about 70%. Other processing creates comparable losses. The Agricultural Research Service of the U.S. Department of Agriculture recently reported that milling and other processing operations of wheat produce a loss of almost 90% of the vitamin E present—in addition to losses of other vitamins.

When you are satisfied that your diet contains sufficient vitamin E from the food as prepared, not just as bought, bear in mind that the addition of other substances to your diet may increase your need for vitamin E. For example, the more polyunsaturated fatty acids in the diet, the more vitamin E is needed. And also bear in mind that the addition of fish liver oils—in food or as medicine—increases the need for vitamin E.

Role of iron.

More particularly, the role of iron in the utilization of vitamin E is often forgotten. Iron is necessary in one type of anemia, hypochromic anemia, in which the amount of hemoglobin is low. But iron also destroys vitamin E!

If you take iron—as a component of multivitamin tables, for example—as well as vitamin E, take them about 12 hours apart. Taking multivitamins in the morning and vitamin E at or after dinner will not expose vitamin E to the deteriorating effect of iron. Remember too that certain foods such as spinach and raisins are also rich in iron. This does not mean to avoid them. But it does mean that if you take a daily vitamin E supplement, you should not take it with a meal that contains iron-rich foods.

Apart from its relation to vitamin E, a large intake

of iron raises a number of problems. Iron is not the safe material it is commonly thought to be.

People who have iron storage disease—though a small percentage of the population is so afflicted—can suffer damage by iron. Those who have a condition (hemochromatosis) in which the tissues are stained with hemoglobin or other blood pigments are also exposed to hazards. The cirrhotic liver of alcoholics (Laennec's cirrhosis) normally has an uphill task to handle the various normal detoxications to support life; iron adds considerably to its burden. In Cooley's anemia (thalassemia), iron may disturb the precarious blood balance by further enlarging the liver, in which organ much of the iron is stored.

The iron heart is a weak heart according to Drs. Buja and Roberts in an article in the August 1971 issue of the *American Journal of Medicine*. Of 135 patients, of which only four had hemochromatosis and 131 had chronic anemia, 19 had deposits of iron in the heart. When there is an iron deposit in the heart, the heart fails. The excess iron in these people came from blood transfusions, and since nearly all of them had anemia, probably from iron medications.

It is entirely possible, though not frequently met, that excessive intake of iron can produce anemia by destroying vitamin E rather than by ministering to it. Making iron available is one thing. Utilizing it is another. For example, people with low stomach acidity (hypochlorhydria) utilize iron only minimally. The administration of vitamin C helps the utilization of iron in normal individuals as well as those with hypochlorhydria.

Further, in figuring the amount of vitamin E consumed in food bear in mind that the older the animal the more vitamin E is necessary to prevent deficiency. It may well be that vitamin E is also indirectly necessary in the metabolism of proteins, vital food substance in aging.

The foods in which vitamin E is naturally present are lettuce and other green leafy vegetables, wheat germ, whole wheat, vegetable oils, fish, meat, eggs, and cereal grains (as well as oils, such as corn oil, derived from cereal grains). This list should be considered in the light of storage, processing, and preparation of these foods. The use of vitamin E supplements, however, removes doubt as to the amount of vitamin E left in foods after destruction through storage, cooking, or processing.

Mark Twain (1835-1910) often delivered himself of a poignant thought without an attempt to be humorous. Since vitamin E is a nutrient necessary to be well-fed, his ingenious observation comes to mind:

> Principles have no real force except when well fed.

CHAPTER 13

Several Other Uses of Vitamin E

It is amazing that a substance such as vitamin E, on which many hundreds of papers have been written and to which four international symposia have been devoted, has been the subject of calumny rather than investigation—defensiveness rather than data. And these attacks have taken place in the face of scientific papers from the United States, Canada, and many parts of Europe. Logic would dictate that vitamin E would be subjected to a long-time and intensive study, similar to the Framingham study on the role of cholesterol in heart disease or to the long-term studies on anticoagulants. (There is an interesting analogy when one considers the intensive studies that were done on anticoagulants in the treatment of thrombosis or after a heart attack. After studies for 20 years there are still two sharply divided camps as to the usefulness of anticoagulants in heart disease, or thrombosis.)

One speculates why vitamin E has not been assessed with the same attention. Can it possibly be due to the first use of vitamin E as an antisterility vitamin in the rat? Can the reason rest in our Puritan ethic where anything that deals with sex is ipso facto "dirty"? (At least there is a consensus that reproduction is somewhat related to sex.)

What better way is there to devitalize those who favor the use of vitamin E than by setting up honest and adequate studies and finding that the effect of vitamin E is a myth? But no such study has ever been done, except for those papers which occasionally appear and report that vitamin E has not been useful or only partially useful in a variety of conditions.

Over the years we have spoken to many cardiologists and specialists in internal medicine to learn their views on vitamin E. Almost invariably their response has been one of the following: *It's-no-good-because-if-it-would-be-everyone-would-be-using-it,* or *it's-no-good-because-I-have-not-heard-a-paper-about-it-at-any-meeting.* One prominent internist, in practice for about 25 years, delivered a gem: "When I was in medical school they never established a need for it because there is no known use for it." He apparently never heard of the anemia of vitamin E deficient babies, though his principal interest is in hematology.

The bizarre point is that the men who condemned vitamin E admittedly had never used it! And in fact, many of the pro or con medical papers written on it often did lack depth.

Dr. Evan V. Shute of London, Ontario, is a giant figure in vitamin E therapy. One may disagree with his enthusiasm and his evangelistic zeal. Yet, had he not persisted in his mission, the likelihood is that vitamin E would have been forgotten and its attributes, such as its role as an antioxidant, though long known might not have been applied to the users recently described. *The Summary* published by the Shute Institute, is a comprehensive source of clinical information, consisting of a digest of papers on vitamin E. Papers with negative findings are also reported therein.

The hundreds of papers published account for the work of almost 800 investigators all over the world. We are logically precipitated into one of the following conclusions: that the investigators who report favorably on vitamin E are either dishonest or incompetent or duped *or they may be right*. Against them are arrayed prominent scientists and clinicians who had done little or no work with vitamin E yet condemn it untested across the board.

Is it perhaps significant that most of the blasts against vitamin E were in the form of editorials rather than scientific papers? If so, what is the significance? The opponents of vitamin E contend that vitamin E is being widely recommended to cure sterility and impotence. Fringe elements in the past had made such claims, but this is no longer true. The most logical procedure to test the truth or falsity of claims made in behalf of vitamin E would be controlled tests in conditions which are amenable to such studies. But controlled studies have not been done by the opponents, except rarely. And the same care and depth should be given to a study on which condemnation is based as is required for a study to show efficacy. In fact, when starting a study one usually does not know what the results will prove. Only when results are in can you assess them.

The following are some of the uses in which vitamin E has been reported with favorable results.

Heart.

Vitamin E has been used both after heart attack and as a prophylactic agent. Admittedly, prophylaxis is difficult to prove. There are many reports on the fibrinolytic effect of vitamin E—that is, in reducing coagulation potential. This would be logical in the treatment of heart attack. Dr. Evan V. Shute also claims that vitamin E is a vasodilator; though others agree on the fibrinolytic activity, they dispute its effect as a vasodilator. (A vasodilator is a substance that causes the inner width of blood vessels to increase.) There is a sizable amount of literature on the use of vitamin E in heart attack. It is significant to note that rats deficient in vitamin E show adverse changes in electrocardiograms.

A number of reports attest to the protection that vitamin E offers against digitalis toxicity. Most of them originated in West Germany.

Arteriosclerosis.

Arteriosclerosis means a hardening of blood vessels, hence reduced elasticity. This condition predisposes one to heart attack. Vitamin E, particularly in conjunction with vitamin B_6 and nicotinic acid, has been favorably reported in the treatment of arteriosclerosis.

Thrombosis.

Since vitamin E has a fibrinolytic effect—it reduces the propensity of blood clotting—it is reasonable to expect it to be useful as a prophylactic agent in clotting formation in the veins, that is, in thrombophlebitis. A considerable body of literature exists for this use, including studies that show that no postoperative thrombosis occurred in patients treated with vitamin E but did occur in those not so treated. Dr. Alton Ochsner has written favorably on the use of vitamin E in postoperative thrombosis.

Menopause.

There are a number of reports in popular journals on the use of vitamin E in the treatment of the symptoms of the menopause. It has been reported to prevent breasts from dropping and libido from declining and to convert a frigid woman into a vigorous and joyful bed companion, especially during the menopause. In men it has been touted to be an aphrodisiac. Apparently none of these claims are true. However, reasonable experiences in the treatment of the menopause by vitamin E with or without estrogens have also been reported in the medical press. But there is no preponderant evidence that vitamin E alone is useful, despite the existence of certain convincing papers. (Incidentally, vitamin E and estrogens are considered to be antagonistic.)

Burns and wounds.

Among the most convincing evidence for the use of vitamin E—as supported by color slides taken by Dr. Evan V. Shute—is the use of vitamin E in burns. When vitamin E is applied to the burned area, few or no contractions are formed, healing proceeds quickly, and in most cases only minimal scars result. Vitamin E was both given internally and applied in the form of an ointment containing 30 I.U. of vitamin E per gram. It would appear that this therapy would also be highly useful for X-ray burns, and many papers in the world literature do describe this use of vitamin E. It would also appear logical to use vitamin E therapy—internal or external—in napalm burns in Viet Nam. But it has never been used for that purpose, according to our knowledge. In fact, it was reported that when offered without charge to one of the relief organizations, it was turned down.

Max Planck (1858–1947), the great German physicist who formulated the quantum theory, put the problem most pointedly:

> A new scientific truth does not triumph by convincing its opponents and making them see the

light, but rather because its opponents eventually die and a new generation grows up that is familiar with it.

CHAPTER 14

Some Aspects of Research on Biological or Biochemical Effects of Vitamin E

The subject of this chapter—biological effects—is virtually the subject of the whole book, because all the effects of vitamin E are biological. We have merely divided the areas into chapters such as the biological effect of vitamin E on malabsorption, on blood, etc.

Research is basically a search for fundamental information. If such information turns out to be positive it is applied to the advantage of man. For example, it was observed in the laboratory that the blood of people, especially infants, deficient in vitamin E undergoes a change when brought into contact with an oxidizing agent, such as hydrogen peroxide. This was a test by which vitamin E deficiency could be detected in man. When the deficiency is found, vitamin E is then used to remedy the deficiency.

The main thrust of basic research is to find out *how* a substance works. Research-oriented scientists are more interested in the discovery of facts than in finding cures. If their approach seems cold-blooded, it is nevertheless absolutely necessary, because if cures are to be found, they must be based on scientific findings.

First, scientists want to know what a substance does. Then they want answers to *how* or *why* the substance works. Research scientists tend to be unconcerned with getting successful examples of the effect of a drug or another substance in improving the health or lives of people. For example, no matter how dramatic the finding—say, if vitamin E works in tuberculosis or venereal disease (it doesn't)—a research scientist remains largely interested in finding out *how* or *why* such effects are experienced. Scientists call this an inquiry into the *mechanism of action*—how a thing works. Then other scientists repeat the work, because a scientific finding must be capable of being duplicated to be taken seriously.

The latest conclave of scientists specifically interested and active in vitamin E research, sponsored by the New York Academy of Sciences, met in New York on December 6 and 7, 1971, so that scientists could share their findings with other scientists. Science grows by sharing information. Sharing fertilizes the work that a scientist does and helps him to decide what corner of the question to explore. For example, sharing information (1) saves researchers from duplicating experiments unnecessarily, (2) often gives researchers an insight into a different phase which needs exploration, (3) often confirms a finding or uncovers flaws in a research study, (4) stimulates a scientist to think more broadly and constructively, (5) reopens and reexamines, in the light of later work, questions that have been considered to be settled. Nothing in science is conclusive—all conclusions are tentative and must be continually tested in the fire of dialectic or scientific dialogue. Above all, results from research help complete the jigsaw puzzle of our knowledge or ignorance.

In fact, to bring this book up to date, a separate section has been added just before publication. That section comprises condensations of the various papers read at that two-day symposium. The authors of the papers that were read and most of the scientists in the audience were among the most illustrious researchers on vitamin E.

How or why?

The mechanism of action by which scientists seek to determine to answer the questions *how* or *why* vitamin E works is not a simple matter to resolve. One of the reasons is that deficiency or deprivation of vitamin E produces, at least in animals, *a greater variety of dysfunctions* than a deficiency of any other vitamin. Hence, depending upon the organ or body system deprived of vitamin E, there is a greater number of manifestations of deficiency. And deficiency expresses itself differently in different organs. In different organs there is a variety of mechanisms of action.

One fundamental belief about the mechanism of action of vitamin E is the Olson hypothesis, which holds that vitamin E probably controls the body synthesis of enzymes by controlling the very basis of life itself—by influencing the nature of the genes that signal the production of enzymes.

Enzymes are substances produced by the body in minute amounts to set off or to keep going a biochemical reaction in the body. They are specific—there is a different enzyme for each different biochemical reaction in the body. One well-known example of an enzyme is pepsin, which digests certain proteins. Since there are thousands—or perhaps tens of thousands—of such reactions going on, it would suggest that there must be approximately an equal number of enzymes at work. This is actually the case—though many enzymes are only predicated or supposed to exist because they have not yet been isolated or studied.

That vitamin E prevents the oxidation of unsaturated

lipids is well known and has been detailed in earlier chapters. We know that vitamin E reduces or prevents oxidation—that largely answers the *how*. But it does not fully answer the *why*.

The effect of vitamin E on oxidation is related to its effect on enzyme action. There is no doubt that when there is a deficiency of vitamin E, some enzyme systems are disturbed. This also largely answers *why*. But here the *how* is not adequately answered because it is not known if vitamin E enters directly into the working of the enzyme matrix and is integrally involved therein, or if it protects some component that enters the enzyme system by being a shield against oxidation, thereby enabling that component to work smoothly. Finding out *how* a substance works is usually an important question in exploring the unknown; but the researcher is not regularly rewarded with answers. It is important to know *how*, because knowing that, one can better design a research plan to produce answers and to apply these answers to improving the health and lives of people.

Where does vitamin E accumulate in the cell? That is a trenchant question, because on that may depend some *how* and *why* answers. If it is adsorbed on the surface of the cell it may be one thing. But it is believed, with good reason, that vitamin E accumulates in the structures inside the cell called mitochondria, microsomes, and the endoplasmic reticulum. When we recall that the mitochondria are the *power-packs* that supply power to enable the cell to function, we begin to realize how intimately vitamin E is involved in the body economy.

It should not be inferred that vitamin E is the most important component of the cell. *No one thing is the most important* component, for the function of the cell can be likened to an orchestra, in which each component or instrument contributes to the smooth working of the whole. The effect of vitamin E may also be likened to financial transactions at a bank—except here the coin is not money but energy, and there are perhaps dozens of other kinds of coins about which we may suspect much but know little. While we do know many of the effects of deficiency, we have considerable areas of ignorance in that facet too, for certain manifestations of chronic disease may be ascribed to other causes or to unknown causes while they may possibly be signs of vitamin E deficiency. One illustration is that in animals vitamin E overcomes some of the results of deficiency but not all of them.

For example, it was shown that although vitamin E overcomes some results of vitamin E deficiency (such as muscular degeneration in chicks), vitamin E alone does not remedy a severe neurological deficiency, namely encephalomalacia, which is a softening of the brain. But vitamin E prevents encephalomalacia from developing.

Another instance where the good effect of vitamin E can be observed is in poisoning, where vitamin E acts as a detoxifying agent. But we do not really know why or how it does so, though some hypotheses have been advanced. As an example, vitamin E reduces the damage to the liver caused by carbon tetrachloride or other similar chlorinated solvents, and it also has been described as protecting the liver from the deterioration caused by alcohol. (Liver disease produced by excessive or even regular intake of alcohol is more common than suspected.)

Another effect of vitamin E related to poisoning is dealt with in the reports concerning digitalis; here, vitamin E has been found to protect against the toxic effect of this drug. Digitalis, a drug used in certain heart conditions, often needs to be given in doses that become toxic, more particularly if digitalis is given regularly over a long period of time. The reason that this toxicity develops is because digitalis is excreted from the body so slowly that it accumulates in the body. This is called cumulative toxicity. Only a few reports on this use of vitamin E have appeared thus far. More work is necessary to learn *if* vitamin E truly protects against digitalis toxicity and if so, *how* or *why*.

Tests for the presence of vitamin E.

One of the difficulties in research with vitamin E lies in questions concerning the tests used to determine its presence, or level, in the body. These are not easily answered questions. Some of the problems:

(1) What should be tested for vitamin E—urine, blood, feces? Excretion usually means that there is enough of a substance in the body, but then again something else may have happened: perhaps the substance has not been absorbed at all, and it is being excreted because the body could not absorb it.

(2) In blood, vitamin E combines with blood protein, as do other substances. It does not prove that the combination with blood proteins is eventually broken and vitamin E is finally absorbed from the combination.

(3) A substance that the body wants to throw off usually is in the form of a breakdown product or an excretion product. When testing for vitamin E in the urine, for example, researchers often test the urine for the presence of breakdown products, measure the amounts, and calculate the amount of vitamin E that the breakdown products represent. But there is often no assurance that the nature and amount of breakdown products are not interfered with and therefore influenced by the presence in the body of another substance. Such another substance, in this instance vitamin K, may give the same breakdown products.

(4) There are different analytical methods—they often do test different breakdown products. For example, by one kind of test one effect—say, the antioxidant effect—is tested, and a different attribute is tested by another test. Thus different tests give different answers and results can be confusing.

(5) Some breakdown products of vitamin E may be the same as those of related substances—say a quinone; then what do the test results really mean?

(6) Other substances—such as selenium, a trace mineral—are believed to affect the role of vitamin E. If this is the case, a test for vitamin E does not reflect the level of vitamin E in the body. Substances may enhance the effect of vitamin E (as selenium possibly does), or they may destroy one of the qualities of vitamin E (as iron does, by reducing its antioxidant effect).

All tests are relative in this area. This is another example of the complexity of vitamin E utilization by the body, and why continued research is necessary. An admission of ignorance is the first step to a learning experience. The words from Epictetus, the Greek Stoic philosopher who lived in the first and second centuries of this era, is highly applicable here:

> It is impossible for anyone to begin to
> learn what he *thinks* he already knows.

Despite these complexities and until they are resolved, it is our belief that it is prudent to take vitamin E in view of its effect on the vital functions detailed in the previous chapters. Since vitamin E has not been reported to be toxic, it becomes a matter of an individual decision to weigh the cost against the possible good.

Supplement

on

The International Conference on Vitamin E and Its Role in Cellular Metabolism, held under the auspices of the New York Academy of Sciences in New York, on December 6 and 7, 1971.

When you are trying to solve a jigsaw puzzle you must be able to put every piece in its proper place to complete the picture. After a good beginning it may suddenly occur to you that pieces from another puzzle have been mixed into the pile of pieces on which you have been working. This would increase your problem and would lead to confusion unless you could separate out the strange pieces.

This is what frequently happens in research. You often get some new information or a new insight.

Such new information or insight can work in different ways: (1) it can be like extra jigsaw pieces and can show you that the direction in which you have been working is not right—you have to start again somewhere down the line; (2) it can solve a problem that has been awaiting solution; (3) it can give you a new insight that may eventually lead to a solution.

Most of the papers presented at the vitamin E conference were supported by grants from government sources, such as divisions of the National Institutes of Health (including the National Institute of Arthritis and

Metabolic Diseases) as well the the U.S. Public Health Service, NASA, the Office of Naval Research; others were supported by the universities with which the participating scientists are connected.

The papers presented at the conference on vitamin E were concerned with a variety of investigations. While they all deal with vitamin E, most explore the basic biological phenomena to determine *why* or *how* vitamin E works, though a few do deal with the use of vitamin E in treatment of disease.

Some of the papers take up the functions of biological membranes, the stability of vitamin E, and how it protects, or stabilizes, membranes. Other papers support or differ with the idea that the way vitamin E works is as a biological antioxidant. How vitamin E works in the cell and how it affects metabolism were considered by other papers (some blood constituents, such as heme, develop differently when there is a deficiency in vitamin E than when there is normal supply). These were followed with presentations on how vitamin E is transported in the human red blood cell and on what the relationship is among the human red blood cell, the fats in that cell, and vitamin E. (An immense number of events can go on in the microscopically sized red blood cell.)

How the polyunsaturated fatty acids are related to the need for vitamin E both in the normal state and in malabsorption was another facet of the overall vitamin E metabolism that was brought out.

In none of the 20 papers at the conference was any intimation made that vitamin E is toxic, even mildly so.

Apparently timed to appear during the vitamin E conference, the *Medical Letter* reported that there is no use for vitamin E in any disease condition. For a number of uses for which vitamin E had been recommended in the past, such as that of an aphrodisiac, this is true. But that publication disclosed no new findings, many of the indications against which it inveighed are no longer considered, and its short (two-page) report was only editorial—no new findings against vitamin E were disclosed. It reported only the negative factors.

It seems to us that any scientific information deserves an unbiased presentation. It is just as objectionable to be nihilistic as it is to beat the drums to promote a nostrum.

In general, vitamin E hinders, impairs, blocks, or impedes some noxious function. For example, it impedes the deteriorating effect of oxygen—as any antioxidant would. In hindering such undesirable action, it helps normal and desirable action to take place. Those activities take place in the cell. But the cell is not the smallest constituent—the submolecular units (the nuclei, membranes, mitochondria) are. This is the reason that studies on the effect of a substance begin with the smallest submolecular units, which collectively make up increasingly larger units, such as cells, organs, tissues, individuals, societies, and environments.

The following are summaries of the papers that were presented at the international conference on vitamin E.

Oxygen and vitamin E.

Breathing oxygen under high pressure was observed to be damaging to red blood cells. The reason is that oxygen, especially in high concentrations and under pressure, causes peroxidation of tissues. This is especially accentuated if there is a deficiency of vitamin E, according to Dr. Charles E. Mengel, a physician and Professor and Chairman of the Department of Medicine of the University of Missouri Medical School in Columbia.

Dr. Mengel's studies demonstrated several things, among which is that peroxidation of lipids can occur in an animal under stress. It had heretofore not been clear whether this peroxidation occurs only in vitro (that is, in chemical models). This work shows that the breakup of red blood cells takes place in the live animal just the same as in the chemical model.

Another finding demonstrated that peroxidation of lipids occurs before the breakup of red blood cells takes place. This means that damage sets in before visual evidence shows it. Saturated fats do not peroxidize—but unsaturated ones do. Dr. Mengel's experiments confirmed this.

An additional point is that cells in tocopherol-deficient animals develop more methemoglobin than do normal cells when challenged with sodium nitrite, which precipitates methemoglobin formation. Methemoglobin does not function to bring oxygen to the tissues—hemoglobin does that. Methemoglobin is what is formed when a person dies of carbon monoxide poisoning.

Stress often precipitates disease. Stresses can be of various kinds, such as exposure to poisoning or to something that disturbs body equilibrium. Oxygen under pressure—or in fact too much oxygenation, especially too much peroxidation—is a stress. Dr. Mengel's work shows how vitamin E protects animals and man against one kind of stress, namely peroxidation.

Dr. Mengel's work reports that in mice deficient in vitamin E, the red blood cells are sensitive to destruction when challenged by too much oxygen, but mice given adequate protection by feeding them vitamin E are not subject to this destruction. In his experiment, using man, he also says that ". . . humans exposed to oxygen under pressure could develop hemolysis"—that is, the destruction of red blood cells.

Depletion and repletion.

How quickly can the body be depleted of vitamin E and how quickly "refilled," or repleted? This is the subject of a paper by Dr. John G. Bieri, physiologist from the Laboratory of Nutrition and Endocrinology of the National Institute of Arthritis and Metabolic Diseases, Bethesda, Maryland. His paper has largely to do with the organs that become depleted of vitamin E and, what is as important, with the rates or the speed with which these depletion-repletion phenomena occur.

At this point we should make some remarks about the overriding importance of speed or slowness at which an event takes place. Throughout this book you will also find reference to such rates.

The rate at which a sequence or an event takes place is most important because timing plays a unique role in most endeavors. For example, in case of a fire the best-equipped fire department is of no use unless it can be instantly alerted and unless it responds at once. Similarly, police protection can become a sorry joke unless a policeman is available to control a criminal incident. In a like vein, though we all know that water can quench thirst, thirst can be quenched only when water is available. Travelers in the desert have died of thirst because water came too late. These are examples where speed is necessary.

But rate also has to do with slowness, and speed can become a threat or danger. For example, the damages that floods do are not due to the rain but to the rapid rate at which water accumulates before it can run off. Similarly, if drinking water comes into a reservoir at a rate more quickly that it is utilized, it can also turn into a flood.

The striking importance of rate is best exemplified by a breaking dam. The amount of water that is in the reservoir is no danger if the rate of outflow is controlled. When a dam breaks, the water engulfs everything in its path, not due to the quantity of water that must be accommodated but due to the fact that all the water becomes available at one time.

Scientists are always concerned about the rate at which an event takes place for similar reasons. When scientists speak of the dynamics, or the kinetics, of a reaction they largely mean the rate—the slowness or the speed—at which a reaction takes place.

Dr. Bieri's study on depletion and repletion concerns the rate at which vitamin E is built up (accumulated) and, commensurately, used up and what happens to the tissues in the interim. Different tissues and organs lose vitamin E at different rates. We do not have a clear picture at this time of all tissues so concerned.

Another thing that complicates the picture is that animals do not lose their vitamin E at a steady rate. For example, when rats are depleted of vitamin E by withholding it from their diet, they quickly lose the large bulk of their body stores of vitamin E in four weeks, but the small remainder is lost much more slowly. Because the rate is uneven, measuring the loss is complicated.

Similarly, all organs do not lose their vitamin E during depletion at the same rate. Both rats and rabbits quickly lose their vitamin E stores in the liver when fed a vitamin E deficient diet, but their muscles lose it much less rapidly. This requires studies of vitamin E loss to be done on each organ separately.

Organs can be divided into two groups pertaining to loss of vitamin E, according to the findings disclosed by Dr. Bieri. Thus, the liver, heart, and blood plasma lose one-half or more of their vitamin E in only one or two weeks, and this rate is accentuated in the organs of animals that need vitamin E most—the young, growing animals.

A considerably slower rate of loss occurs in the other group of organs, namely in the testes, fat, and muscle.

There is a rate within a rate. Losses in all organs of animals on a vitamin E deficient diet are greatest during the first few weeks and slower after that. This means that if damage occurs it takes place relatively quickly, even though the results of the damage are not quickly apparent. The same results were also found in monkeys. Dr. Bieri believes that a similar situation occurs in man.

What happens when a vitamin E depleted animal is again fed vitamin E to replenish or accumulate the stores of the vitamin? That is an interesting story.

It takes much longer for the animal body to accumulate because by and large the rate of repletion is slower than that of depletion. And the rate is not even. The body accumulates vitamin E at a faster rate after a lag period.

This corresponds to the general observation that vitamin E is a sluggish vitamin—it acts slowly. It is also a sluggish antioxidant. While the rate of loss is not rapid, the rate of accumulation is even slower.

This would suggest that it is not good for an animal to get into a vitamin E deficient state. The matter becomes all the more important when seen in the light of the remark of Dr. M. K. Horwitt, of the St. Louis University School of Medicine, that vitamin E "obviously has a requirement." While he thinks many people who do not need it as a supplement are taking it, nevertheless, says Dr. Horwitt, "You cannot live without it. The question is do you have enough or don't you?"

Dr. Bieri's final finding from his experiments: after several weeks on a vitamin E deficient diet, which was not supplemented later with vitamin E, there was greater blood destruction, greater creatine excretion, and later, greater degeneration of the testes than in animals not depleted. And more particularly, after depletion, he found that merely giving a greater amount of vitamin E did not mean a greater recovery. In customary scientific language, Dr. Bieri reports that in most tissues, including blood plasma, "a linear relationship was found between the tissue concentration of [vitamin E] and the *log* of the dietary alpha-tocopherol." This means that you do not get twice the effect by giving twice as much vitamin E.

Drug metabolism.

Many drugs taken into the body would be poisonous unless they were detoxified by the liver. In this detoxication a number of enzymes or enzyme systems are involved. Certain structures (called microsomes) in the liver, that marvelous chemical factory of the body, detoxify various drugs by changing them.

The liver changes different drugs in different ways to make them less toxic or more potent. One of the several ways the liver changes drugs in the process of detoxification is called hydroxylation. Hydroxylation is the function of putting a hydroxyl radical, referred to as an *OH* radical, on a molecule.

In a paper on the relation of vitamin E to drug hydroxylation by microsomes, Dr. Mary P. Carpenter, biochemist from the Oklahoma Medical Research Foundation and the University of Oklahoma Health Sciences Center, Oklahoma City, postulated that vitamin E deficiency in animals depresses microsomal drug metabolism by reducing hydroxylation and that, conversely, the administration of vitamin E increases liver microsomal drug metabolism of certain drugs. It was also her finding that vitamin E as well as another antioxidant, with the jawbreaking name of N, N'-diphenyl-p-phenylene-diamine, commonly called DPDD, can replace vitamin E in preventing a number of vitamin E deficiency symptoms, but it does not replace the effect of vitamin E on microsomal hydroxylation.

What this means is that such basic research puts down fundamentals in the area in which many of the basic properties of vitamin E are postulated.

Newborn babies' anemia.

The role of vitamin E in anemia of premature infants was discussed by two physicians, Dr. Samuel Gross and Dr. David N. Melhorn, associate professor and assistant professor, respectively, of the Department of Pediatrics of the Case Western Reserve University, Cleveland. They reaffirmed the effect of vitamin E in the alarming type of anemia that threatens the lives of prematurely born infants. They assessed the role of vitamin E and its relation to iron administration during the first four months of life of premature infants.

One conclusion, among others reached by them, is that iron, which is given to these infants to treat the anemia, actually exaggerates the blood-destroying (hemolytic) process. When iron is administered with vitamin E, absorption of both iron and vitamin E is impaired, and the younger the premature infant the worse the impairment of absorption. In their study, which continued over three years, they studied 234 such premature infants. The birth weight of these infants ranged from somewhat less than 3½ pounds (1500 grams) to somewhat less than 4½ pounds (2000 grams).

Their work once again confirms material described earlier in this book—namely, that a deficiency in vitamin E decreases the survival of red blood cells in premature infants and that the anemia due to vitamin E deficiency is caused by lipid peroxidation of the membranes of the red blood cells.

Animal anemia.

Another presentation on the role of vitamin E in anemia concerned certain species of animals. A fine basic paper on that subject by Dr. Coy D. Fitch, physician from the Department of Internal Medicine of the St. Louis University School of Medicine, reminded the participants that while it is now generally acknowledged that anemia is one of the diseases induced by vitamin E deficiency, two aspects of this type of anemia are sometimes forgotten. The first aspect is that the reason (the *why*) for anemia associated with vitamin E deficiency may differ from species to species of animal. The second is that in such animals such anemia can be produced by (1) blood loss, as in hemorrhage, (2) oxidant hemolysis, as when blood destruction occurs due to lipid peroxidation of the red blood cell, and (3) ineffective erythropoiesis, as when new blood formation is impaired.

The first cause of such anemia—blood loss due to hemorrhage—occurs in poultry deficient in vitamin E. Blood leaking into the tissues is a condition associated with exudative diathesis, one of the symptoms of vitamin E deficiency.

The second cause of such anemia—namely oxidant hemolysis—is demonstrated when blood of vitamin E deficient rodents is brought into contact with an oxidizing agent, such as a dilute solution of hydrogen peroxide. (This test, incidentally, also shows blood disturbance due to factors other than vitamin E deficiency, such as sickle-cell anemia.)

The third cause of vitamin E deficient anemia is defective blood formation. This condition develops in monkeys and, though long in developing, is fatal. But if a large dose for monkeys, say 100 milligrams, of alpha-tocopherol is given even during the long state of vitamin E deficiency, ". . . the response of the anemic, vitamin E deficient monkey is dramatic and complete."

Dr. Fitch, however, makes the comparison by stating that adding other blood-forming materials such as iron, folic acid, and vitamin B_{12} ". . . does not affect the anemia of vitamin E deficiency in the monkey." And he pleads for further research on the *why* of this mechanism.

Free radical scavenger.

That dietary vitamin E has a regulatory effect on lipid peroxidation or on other degradation of lipids in the normal course of certain steps in energy metabolism, steps which are necessary to sustain life, was established by Drs. Paul B. McCay, Peter M. Pfeifer, and William H. Stipe, biochemists at the Oklahoma Medical Research Foundation and the University of Oklahoma Health Sciences Center, Oklahoma City.

During this work they demonstrated that vitamin E from the tissues is changed into a compound that by and large impedes oxidation. Here again it was brought out that under certain circumstances the ". . . higher content of alpha-tocopherol in the erythrocyte [red blood cell] membrane apparently provides the margin of radical trapping required to prevent hemolysis." This means that free radicals, as outlined in Chapter 3, need to be trapped because they peroxidize lipids, including the polyunsaturated fatty acids. Vitamin E is an antioxidant and acts as such a free radical trap.

In the process whereby free radicals promote peroxidative destruction of lipids, vitamin E, which acts as a shield, is itself partially used up when this destructive reaction begins. Dr. McCay and associates conclude that, since vitamin E is itself partially consumed, ". . . elevating the level of alpha-tocopherol in these membranes delays the onset of the attack on the polyunsaturated fatty acids" in the tissues. And they affirm that "when the level of alpha-tocopherol is sufficiently decreased, attack on the membrane polyunsaturated fatty acids of the membrane then commences."

These researchers agree with the notion generally advanced regarding the deposition of pigments (such as lipofuscin), that the major function of vitamin E is that of a free radical scavenger. They clearly summarize their presentation with the limitations that are well known: "while direct evidence still has to be obtained it appears feasible that the effects of tocopherol deficiency disease are consequences of damage caused by radicals"—which are associated with the activity of the enzyme systems they studied.

Polyunsaturates and vitamin E.

It is generally believed at present that the greater the intake of vegetable oils containing polyunsaturated fatty acids, the greater the need for vitamin E. This view is challenged by Dr. F. C. Jager, biochemist of Unilever Research, Vlaardingen, Holland. Dr. Jager believes that much more polyunsaturated fatty acid is needed than heretofore believed before the body needs an increase of vitamin E.

This is a matter of quantity and does not affect the general utility of vitamin E. Whether Dr. Jager's views and calculations will be found to be correct can be largely determined in the future. He may well turn out to be right. But until that time, it is safer to hold to the currently established view, which is that the greater the intake of polyunsaturated fatty acids, the greater the need of vitamin E, in order to prevent vitamin E deficiency.

Vitamin E requirements and polyunsaturates.

But Dr. Lloyd A. Witting, biochemist from the nutrition research laboratories of the Elgin State Hospital, Elgin, Illinois, does hold that the vitamin E requirement is influenced by polyunsaturated fatty acids. He stated that since vitamin E is partially used up by the polyunsaturated fatty acids in membranes, the body needs extra amounts supplied from the outside—in other words, as the tissue lipid content is increased, there is an increased need for vitamin E. He believes that increased destruction of vitamin E is related to a high polyunsaturated fatty acid content in the tissues.

This is not a simple equation. Dr. Witting states wisely that different polyunsaturated fatty acids generate different vitamin E requirements, depending on the degree of unsaturation of the polyunsaturated fatty acids. The degree is not a simple matter to determine, and just loading up with huge amounts of vitamin E does not give the answer. To use one example to illustrate the point: at least in the rat, says Dr. Witting, during "simultaneous depletion of vitamin E and polyunsaturated fatty acids, vitamin E is depleted faster than polyunsaturated fatty acids."

Most of the vitamin E requirement, he pointed out, is to "quench free-radical initiated peroxidative chain reactions in membrane lipids"—on which idea there is general agreement.

The accumulation of the so-called age pigment, or senile pigment (such as ceroid or lipofuscin), which seems to be associated with vitamin E deficiency, was also briefly considered by Dr. Witting.

Cystic fibrosis and vitamin E.

Cystic fibrosis of the pancreas was referred to in the

chapter on malabsorption in this book. Cystic fibrosis is an inherited disease that affects infants, children, and young adults. Its symptoms, though found in several body systems, are largely characterized by chronic disease of the lungs in which an accumulation of viscid mucus interferes with respiration and by deficiencies in the function of the pancreas and of the sweat glands. The perspiration is unusually high in salts. In cystic fibrosis there is a considerably reduced level of vitamin E in the blood plasma.

A paper discussing polyunsaturated fatty acids and vitamin E levels in patients with cystic fibrosis was presented by Drs. Barbara A. Underwood, Carolyn R. Denning, and M. Navab, of the Institute of Human Nutrition and Department of Pediatrics of the College of Physicians and Surgeons, Columbia University, New York. They found that only patients who were given a vitamin E supplement had a normal level of vitamin E in blood and those who did not receive supplemental vitamin E had markedly reduced levels of vitamin E in blood. In fact, it is known that in cystic fibrosis there is customarily a low level of vitamin E in the blood.

This does not mean that vitamin E is a cure for cystic fibrosis or that no other substances are involved therein. But it does mean that the supplementation with vitamin E raises the vitamin E in the tissues of people with cystic fibrosis, whose vitamin E level is well known to be low.

Biologic membranes.

Biologic membranes have two functions: (1) to make walls for the cells and (2) to provide a place where pockets of enzymes can hang, said Dr. J. A. Lucy, physiologist and biochemist from the School of Medicine of the Royal Free Hospital of the University of London. In proper "scientese" it comes out that the functions of membranes is "the compartmentalization of cells and the provision of structural framework for the attachment of enzymes"—as put by Dr. Lucy.

That these two functions are vitally important is clear. Were the human body to develop (if it could) without cells, there would be no differentiation into organs. Each organ accomplishes its separate task to provide the celestial harmony of functions that the human body represents.

Dr. Lucy suggests that membrane integrity is preeminently indispensable—with which no one can disagree. And he posits the idea that in vitamin E deficiency abnormalities occur in the structure of membranes—abnormalities that result in a failure of one or both of the membrane functions.

This means that in vitamin E deficiency cell walls deteriorate, and places on which enzyme packs hang disappear. It may sound trivial, but if these things happen results can be grave.

Vitamin E may have functions other than that of an antioxidant against polyunsaturated fatty acids, speculates Dr. Lucy. One such may be that vitamin E acts as an antioxidant for proteins containing selenium. He proposes that vitamin E may stabilize those membranes that contain many polyunsaturated fatty acids—and he suggests a physico-chemical basis by which this possibly takes place.

The thrust of his thesis is that while vitamin E is necessary in preserving the integrity of membranes, it probably acts in a different way than a simple, or ordinary, antioxidant does.

How much vitamin E?

The amount of vitamin E recommended for daily use varies in different countries: 10 milligrams in Switzerland, 5 to 30 milligrams in Germany, 20 to 30 milligrams in the United States. This stimulated two British physicians, Drs. M. S. Losowsky and J. Kelleher of the Department of Medicine of the University of Leeds and the St. James Hospital of Leeds, to discuss the intake and absorption of vitamin E.

Measuring the amounts of vitamin E in the daily diet of a group of hospital patients as well as of several young healthy people in England, they found that about 50% of the diets were too low in vitamin E. This was despite the fact that the diets were otherwise nutritionally suitable. As a result, Drs. Losowsky and Kelleher believe that, at least in Britain, many people do not get enough vitamin E.

Despite their finding that the normal individuals had reasonable though low vitamin E levels, they say that vitamin E cannot be considered in the light of the polyunsaturated fatty acid intake, as the latter increases the need for vitamin E. In their study the normal individuals who had a low but not deficient level of vitamin E were those who also had a low intake of polyunsaturated fatty acids—which may explain why with a low vitamin E intake no deficiencies were shown.

This reaffirms the relation between polyunsaturated fatty acids and vitamin E— the more of the former in the dietary intake, the more of the latter is necessary.

Paradoxically, as to absorption, they found that the larger the dose of vitamin E the smaller the proportion (or percentage) but not the amount of absorption. They also reported that fat absorption parallels vitamin E absorption.

Vitamin E as an antioxidant.

A long paper, with over 100 references, attacking the theory that vitamin E works as an antioxidant was given by Dr. J. Green, biochemist of the Nutritional Research Center in Beecham Research Laboratories,

Surrey, England. Full of drama and bibliographic references, Dr. Green did not necessarily question that vitamin E has an effect on the various conditions in which it has been described to work. He merely disputed the belief that it works by overcoming peroxidation. In sum, he did not believe that any of the effects of vitamin E work according to an antioxidant theory.

Does he have a theory of his own to counter the antioxidant theory? Yes and no; he quotes instead the works of several other investigators suggesting that vitamin E works because it facilitates the transport of amino acids across the membranes of the intestine. Other reports which Dr. Green believes may bear study have different proposals—for example, that in vitamin E deficiency there may be a defect of collagen metabolism or that vitamin E stabilizes selenium.

The vigor of his attack on the antioxidant theory—especially when he did not disagree with the classical effects reported by various laboratories—created considerable discussion. But on one point there was unison: that continued research is imperative on *how* or *why* vitamin E works.

New insight.

Dr. M. K. Horwitt, of the Department of Biochemistry, St. Louis University School of Medicine, has been in the forefront of vitamin E research for about 20 years. But the nature of science is such that if new evidence or insight is presented, a scientist with integrity will change his views, even if long held.

Thus, Dr. Horwitt now thinks that the ways the level of vitamin E nutrition is expressed are not adequate and he suggests remedies.

The level of vitamin E in the blood serum depends in great part, Dr. Horwitt holds, on the rise and fall of the lipids in blood serum. These lipids include cholesterol, triglycerides, and phospholipids.

And the level of these lipids is influenced in turn by genetic or dietary factors, as well as the physiologic state.

This is a comparatively new concept. It does not have anything to do with the effect that vitamin E may have, but deals primarily with the question of how to consider the various other factors in the blood (such as the lipid level) when expressing the vitamin E level in the blood.

Free radicals.

An eminent researcher on vitamin E who is also a prolific writer is Dr. A. L. Tappel, biochemist at the University of California at Davis. References to his work have been made in many parts of this book. Dr. Tappel is an expert in the peroxidation of lipids by free radicals and in the role of vitamin E in impeding the damage done by free radicals.

The thrust of Dr. Tappel's argument, in the highly complex subject of how vitamin E suppresses lipid peroxidation, is that vitamin E reacts by breaking the chain that leads to peroxidation. He explains further that peroxidation of the lipids in membranes produces damaging products—and vitamin E breaks the vicious cycle. Among these damaging products are the lipofuscin-like (ceroid) pigments discussed in detail in this book. His contribution to the vitamin E conference, one of the longer papers, went into considerable detail on the mechanics of the chemical changes involved. He pointed out that vitamin E shows only modest antioxidant activity, and that "vitamin E and other chain-breaking antioxidants reach their maximum effectiveness at similar concentrations." There are several antioxidants that suppress lipid peroxidation. But none of them has been as extensively studied as vitamin E.

Cells and vitamin E action.

There are many levels of structure. But they all have one common denominator—the cell. Organs are composed of different groups of cells.

Dr. Klaus Schwarz, physician-researcher in the Department of Biological Chemistry of the School of Medicine of the University of California at Los Angeles and the U.S. Veterans Hospital in Long Beach, is one of the proponents of the selenium theory of vitamin E activity. His contribution at the vitamin E conference dealt with how vitamin E works. He stated that while vitamin E prevents respiratory decline of the cells, it does not do so by antioxidant action. He concluded that vitamin E has both a direct and an indirect method of action and that both these methods of action take place alongside other highly complex events that go on in the cells (in which the role of certain enzymes figures prominently).

Vitamin E, hormones, and blood.

Vitamin E as a regulator of the synthesis of heme and hemoprotein—blood components—was briefly described by Dr. P. P. Nair, biochemist at the Sinai Hospital of Baltimore. With his associates he discovered that vitamin E is remedial in a rare but serious condition, porphyria, previously discussed in this book.

Dr. Nair speculated that "the effect of vitamin E as a biological antioxidant could arise indirectly as a result of a depression" of scavenging of peroxides.

Other researchers from the same institution described several other different functions of vitamin E. Dr. David Solomon, physician at both the Sinai Hospital and the

Johns Hopkins University School of Medicine, found that deficiency in vitamin E in experimental animals leads to a change in the excretion of certain hormones (specifically, 17-ketosteroids and pregnandiol), which shows an upset in the hormonal system. When he used vitamin E in six women with cysts in the breasts, four showed marked improvement.

A highly esoteric investigation by Dr. Judith W. Hauswith, a biochemist of the Department of Medicine of the Sinai Hospital investigated the place in the microscopic cell where vitamin E probably acts.

Dr. Priscilla I. Caasi of the same department found that vitamin E deficiency, "results in a reduced capacity to synthesize heme," an important blood element.

Epilogue

What is the *bottom line* resulting from the conclave of scientists at the New York Academy of Sciences conference on vitamin E?

There are several such bottom lines.

As disclosed by the conference, one is that vitamin E does play a role in diseases of animals and also in some diseases of man. These apparently would not have been improved without vitamin E.

Another includes the finding that there are other materials—such as selenides (selenium derivatives), DPDD, and butylated hydroxytoluene—that can replace some of the functions of vitamin E. Note: most are not generally safe to take—do not go off experimentally or you may go off the cliff.

A third is that scientists differ on *how* vitamin E works—and often on *why*. Vitamin E may work as a biological antioxidant, and the camp of adherents of this idea is large; another camp, having a different view, does not accept the antioxidant theory but does not dispute the effectiveness of vitamin E in certain conditions. Either camp may prove to be right—only time can decide. And it may possibly turn out when a new hypothesis is put forth and eventually is solidly proved, that both camps are wrong.

The final bottom line, on which all scientists agree, is that much more research on vitamin E is necessary and that this research is worth the time and money that it takes.

But more than time and money are necessary to overcome problems and to solve mysteries. The ferment to fruition is hope and devotion.

In the human condition hope and devotion have currently lost much of their vogue despite their eternal power and presence. This concept was expressed with great insight by Dr. John J. Putnam, a renowned physician who thrived in Boston in the latter part of the 19th century:

> No argument is needed to show what transforming power the mind can exert. The energy set free by the magic agencies of hope, courage, desperation, fanaticism, or by the enthusiasm for a great cause, may reveal the possession of a force undreamed of, or so husband the resources of the body as to keep the flame of life burning for a time when the oil seems exhausted.*

* "Not the Disease Only, But Also the Man," *Boston Medical and Surgical Journal* 141:53, 1899.

Glossary

arteriosclerosis	hardening of the arteries
atherosclerosis	a pathological condition in which there is a deposition of fatty material, usually cholesterol-like, in the walls of arteries
blood plasma	blood, especially the fluid portion, which contains the blood corpuscles and fibrinogen (the clotting component)
blood serum	a clear liquid, from blood or plasma, from which the suspended corpuscles and clotting factors have been removed by clotting
celiac disease	a nontropical sprue-like disease
ceroid	a pigment deposited in the tissues, usually as the organism ages
collagen	gristle; a protein-like material which is one of the components of connective tissue

creatine	a sulfur-containing amino acid
creatinuria	the presence of creatine in urine
cystic fibrosis of the pancreas	a disease of the pancreas in which there is a combination of sacs of fluid with formation of fibrous tissue, which prevents the normal functioning of the pancreas
deficiency	when referring to vitamin deficiency denotes an intake of a vitamin that is less than adequate to maintain health; the appearance of symptoms signaling such deficiency.
encephalomalacia	softening of the brain
endoplasm	the central, innermost part of a cell—distinguished from the outer part of a cell (ectoplasm)
endoplast	cell nucleus
exudative diathesis	a combination of swollen glands, eczema, and edema
gluten	a component of wheat flour
hematocrit	a measure of the volume of blood corpuscles
heme	(formerly called hematin) a protoporphyrin pigment, containing iron, that occurs in hemoglobin as well as in other cells and is involved in carrying oxygen to the tissues
hemolysis	the destruction of red blood cells
intermittent claudication	lameness that appears on walking

lipids — a group of substances characterized by some properties of fats

lipofuscin — a brown, fat-containing pigment

malabsorption — a disorder of intestinal digestion characterized by the inability to absorb fat or other nutrients

metabolism — the sum of events or happenings that go on in the body relating to the utilization of food, conversion into energy, and other changes that support health and life itself

microsome — a minute granular structure in cells, (especially in the liver) that contains enzymes

muscular dystrophy — a progressive condition characterized by wasting of muscles

oxidation — the process of taking on oxygen

pancreatitis — inflammation of the pancreas

peripheral vascular disease — a condition in which the circulation of the blood in the legs is impeded

reduction — the process of losing oxygen

respiratory — related to breathing

reticulum — a network of tissue, usually in the cell

sprue — a disease in which diarrhea, ulcers of the gastrointestinal tract, and other digestive anomalies are prominent—tropical and nontropical

symptom — a happening which suggests that there is a departure from normal

	functioning; a complaint regarding that happening
syndrome	a group of symptoms related to a particular disease
thrombophlebitis	development of clots in the veins of the leg

Bibliography

Baker, E. M., Hammer, D. C., March, S. C., Tolbert, B. M., & Canham, J. E. Science 173; 827; Aug. 27, 1971

Bennet, M. J. Paper read at the Meeting of the Federation of American Society of Experimental Biology, April 1966

Binder, H. J., & Shapiro, H. M. N. E. J. Med. 273; 1290; Dec. 9, 1965

Braunstein, H. Gastroenterology 40; 224; Feb. 1961

Buja, L. M. & Roberts, W. C. Am. J. Med. 51; 209; Aug. 1971

Bunnell, R. H., Keating, J., Quaresimo A., & Parman, G. K. Am. J. Clin. Nutr. 17; 1; July 1965

Chem. & Eng. News, June 29, 1970, "Vitamins A & E Maintain Lung Health"

Christensen, F., Dam, H., & Gortner, R. A. Acta Physiol. Scandinav. 36; 82; 1956

DiLuzio, N. R. Given at Annual Meeting of ACS, April 1971. Abstract in Modern Medicine, p. 80, June 14, 1971

Dinning, J. S. Paper read at Meeting of Fed. of Amer. Soc. Exp. Biol., April 1963

Evans, H. A. & Burr, G. O. JAMA 88; 1462; 1927
JAMA 88; 1587; 1927

Evans, J. W. & Bishop, K. S. Science 56; 650-651; Dec. 8, 1922

Goldbloom, R. B. Can. Med. Assn. J. 82; 1114; May 28, 1960
Goldstein, B. D. Science 169; 605; Aug. 7, 1970
Gross, S., & Guilford, M. V. J. Nutrition 100, 1099; Sept. 1970
György, P. Science 108; 716; 1948 Proc. Soc. Exp. Biol. & Med. 74; 411; 1950. Am. J. Physiol. 168; 414; 1952
Harris P. L., Hardenbrook, E. G., Dean, F. P., Cusack, E. R., & Jensen, J. L. Proc. Soc. Exp. Biol. & Med. 107; 381; 1961
Harris, R. S. Vitamins & Hormones 20; 603; 1962
Helwing, H-P, Hochrein, H., & Hennersdorf, G. Arch. Pharmak. & Exp. Path. 203; 220; 1968
Herting, D. C. Am. J. Clin. Nutr. 19; 210; 1966
Herting, D. C., & Drury, E. E. Federation Proceedings 28; No. 2; March-April 1969
Hillman, R. W. Am. J. Clin. Nutr. 5; 597; 1957
Horwitt, M. K. Borden's Rev. Nutrition Res. 22; 1; 1961
Horwitt, M. K. Am. J. Clin. Nutr. 8; 451; July-Aug. 1960
Horwitt, M. K. Vitamins & Hormones, p. 541, Academic Press, N.Y., 1962
Kingsbury, K. J., & Ward, R. J. Brit. Med. J. 1; 1958; 1961
Krumdiek, C. L. JAMA; 251; 1652; March 8, 1971
Loesel, L. S., Schnitzer B., & Herting, D. C. Paper read at Meeting of Int. Acad. of Path., March 11, 1969, 58th Annual Meeting, San Francisco
Majaj, A. S., et al. Am. J. Clin. Nutr. 12; 374; 1963
Manhold, J. H. "Effects of Social Stress on Oral and Other Bodily Tissues" delivered at the 48th general meeting of the International Association of Dental Research, March 18, 1970
Menzel, D. B. Ann. Rev. Phclogy. 10; 379; 1970
Nair, P. P., Mezey, E., Murti, H. S., Quartner, J., & Mendeloff, A. I. Arch. Int. Med. 128; 411; Sept. 1971
Nitkowsky, H. M., Hsu, K. S., & Gordon, H. H. Vitamins & Hormones, p. 559, Academic Press, N.Y., 1962
Nitkowsky, H. M., Tildon, J. T., Levin, S., & Gordon, H. H. Am. J. Clin. Nutr. 10; 368; May 1962
Ochsner, A. N.E.J.Med. 271; 211; 1964
Passawater, R. J., & Welker, P. A. American Lab., pp. 21-26, May 1971
Pryor, W. A. Scientific Amer. 223; 70; Aug. 1970
Pryor, W. A. Chem & Engineering News, June 7, 1971

Raychaudhuri, C., & Desai, I. D. Science 173; 1028; Sept. 10, 1971

Ritchie, J. H., Fish, M. B., McMasters, V., & Grossman, M. N. E. J. Med. 279; 1185; 1968

Roehm, J. N., Hadley, J. G., & Menzel, D. B. Arch. Int. Med. 128; 88; July 1971; also Chem. & Engineering News, June 29, 1970

Roels, O. A. Knowledge of Vitamin E—in Present Knowledge in Nutrition, 3rd Edition, The Nutrition Foundation, N.Y. 1967

Sahud & Cohen. Lancet 1; 937; 1971

Schroeder, H. A. Am. J. Clin. Nutr. 24; 562; May 1971

Schroeder, H. A., Frost, D. V., & Balassa, J. J. J. Chron. Dis. 23; 227; 1970

Schwarz, K., & Foltz, C. M. Fed. Proc. 19; 421; 1960

Senior, R. M., Wessler, S., & Avioli, L. V. JAMA 217; 1373; Sept 6, 1971

Serrill, J., et al. Aerospace Med. 42; 436; 1971

Shute, E. V., et al. Surg. Gynec. & Obstet. 86; 1; 1948

Storey, P. B. J. Psychosomat. Res. 13; 175-182; 1969

Tappel, A. L. Geriatrics 23; 97; Oct. 1968

Tappel, A. L., Zalkin, H., & Knapp, M. S. Paper read at (Chicago) Annual Meeting of the Federation of Amer. Soc. of Exp. Biol. April 11, 1960

Toone, W. M. Angiology 18; 409; July 1967

Towbin, A. JAMA 217; 1207; Aug. 30, 1971

Van Vleet, J. F. Am. J. Pathol. 52; 1067; 1968

Williams, H. T. G., Fenna, D., & Macbeth, R. A. Surg. Gynec. & Obstet. 132; April 1971

Williams, R. J. Perspectives in Biol. & Med. 14; 608; Summer 1971

Witting, L. A. Progr. Chem. Fats Other Lipids 9; 519; 1970

Index